Dynamic Light Scattering Spectroscopy of the Human Eye

Jeffrey N. Weiss

Dynamic Light Scattering Spectroscopy of the Human Eye

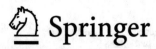 Springer

Jeffrey N. Weiss
The Healing Institute
Margate, FL, USA

ISBN 978-3-031-06626-9   ISBN 978-3-031-06624-5   (eBook)
https://doi.org/10.1007/978-3-031-06624-5

This Springer imprint is published by the registered company Springer Nature Switzerland AG
The registered company address is: Gewerbestrasse 11, 6330 Cham, Switzerland

For the patients that have allowed me the privilege to serve.

Preface

Retinal disease is a common cause of visual loss in the developed countries. A major difficulty in retinal research is the lack of a sensitive, noninvasive, and quantitative method to objectively determine the functional ability of the retina. Visual acuity and visual field testing are subjective methods and depend on patient response. Fundus photography, fluorescein angiography, and ocular coherence tomography (OCT) are imaging tests which are indirectly related to functional ability and detect retinal damage late in the degenerative process. Electrophysiologic testing is difficult to perform and evaluate. The early detection of retinal damage at the microscopic level when it is still potentially reversible is a prerequisite for the development of potential cures. The early detection of the effectiveness of treatment allows for better and more effective therapies.

Dynamic Light Scattering (DLS), also known as Photon Correlation Spectroscopy (PCS), or quasi-elastic light scattering (QLS), is a technique which measures the scattered light intensity fluctuations resulting from the thermal random motion (Brownian motion) of particles.

This technique has been used to predict the development of cataract formation in rabbits, detect the development and monitor diabetes mellitus in humans, assess the quality of treatments for wet macular degeneration, and the effectiveness of retinal stem cell surgery. The results demonstrated the utility of DLS to noninvasively quantitate subtle changes at the molecular level.

This book will present the background, history, and future of utilizing Dynamic Light Scattering Spectroscopy (DLS) to make measurements from the eye.

Parkland, FL, USA   Jeffrey N. Weiss

Contents

Chapter 1
Ocular Anatomy

How Does the Eye Work?

Simplistically, the eye has been compared to a camera. The cornea and lens of the eye focus light onto the retina, or the "film in the camera." The optic nerve carries the image to the brain, like a cable to a computer monitor, for interpretation (Fig. 1.1).

Figure 1.2 depicts what your physician sees when looking into your left eye with an ophthalmoscope. The optic disc is the circular object on the left, the macula is the reddish structure in the middle of the photograph. The fovea is the slightly clearer object in the center of the macula. The retinal veins are slightly wider and deeper in color than the arteries. In your right eye, the location of the optic disc and the macula would be reversed, the optic nerve would be on the right side of the photo, and the macula on the left side.

Figure 1.3 is a picture of an optical coherence tomogram (OCT), a diagnostic test which demonstrates a cross-sectional view of the retina.

The human retina consists of ten layers. Starting inside the eye, moving backwards or posteriorly the layers are:

1. Inner limiting membrane: basement membrane consisting of Muller cells.
2. Nerve fiber layer: this layer represents the axons, similar to "wires" coming from the ganglion layer below, that enter the optic nerve and transmit their messages to the brain.
3. Ganglion cell layer: this layer contains the nuclei of the ganglion cells and some amacrine cells.
4. Inner plexiform layer: this layer contains the connection, or synapse between the bipolar cell axons and the connection structures, or dendrites of the ganglion and amacrine cells.
5. Inner nuclear layer: it contains the nuclei and the cell bodies of the bipolar cells.
6. Outer plexiform layer: the ends of the rods and cones (the photoreceptors) make synapses, or connections with the dendrites of the bipolar cells.

J. N. Weiss, *Dynamic Light Scattering Spectroscopy of the Human Eye*,
https://doi.org/10.1007/978-3-031-06624-5_1

Fig. 1.1 The human eye

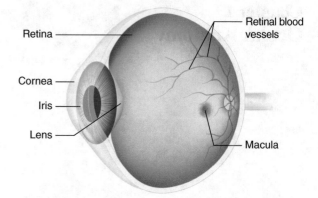

Retina

Cornea

Iris

Lens

Retinal blood vessels

Macula

Fig. 1.2 Physician's view of left eye through the ophthalmoscope

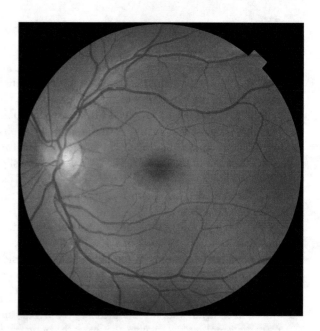

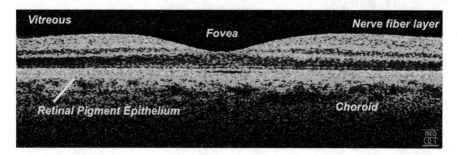

Vitreous

Nerve fiber layer

Fovea

Retinal Pigment Epithelium

Choroid

Fig. 1.3 Optical coherence tomogram

7. Outer nuclear layer: it contains the cell bodies of the rods and cones.
8. External limiting membrane: this membrane separates the inner segment of the photoreceptors from their cell nucleus.
9. Photoreceptor layer: this layer contains the rods and cones.
10. Retinal pigment epithelium: this is a layer of cells.

Figure 1.4 is a cross-section of the retinal anatomy. The retina and optic nerve are part of the central nervous system (CNS) and are the only parts of the CNS that can be directly visualized. The image you see is not just displayed on the retina; it is processed in the retina. In this respect, the retina is more like a computer than a simple film in a camera.

Figure 1.5 is a stylized cross-sectional view of the retina. Light passes from the left (the front of the retina) through the nerve layers to reach the rods and the cones on the far right. A chemical change occurs in the rods and cones which sends a signal to the nerves. The signal is processed by the bipolar and horizontal cells (yellow layer) to the amacrine cells and ganglion cells (purple layer), and then to the optic nerve fibers which go to the brain.

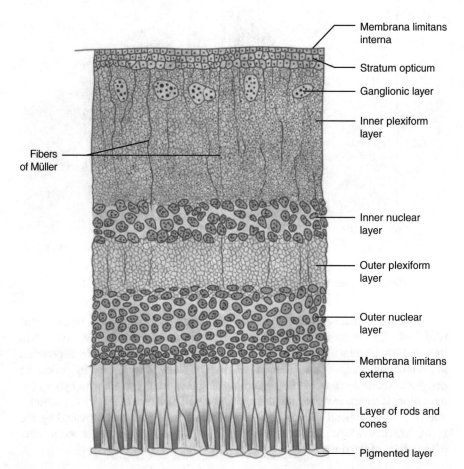

Fig. 1.4 Cross-section of the retinal anatomy

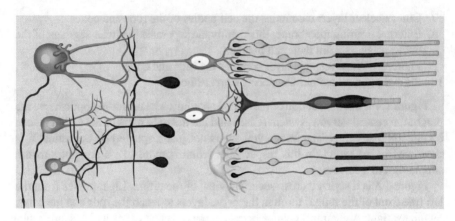

Fig. 1.5 Stylized cross sectional view of the retina

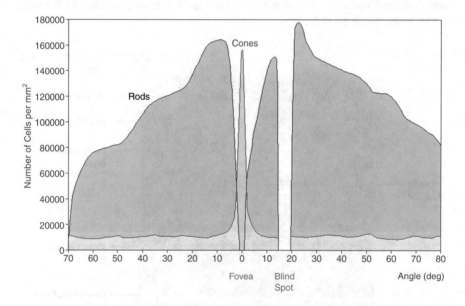

Fig. 1.6 Number of retinal cells per mm²/angle in degrees

The retina contains approximately 7 million cones, and 75–150 million rods (Fig. 1.6). The cones are utilized in daylight, and for color vision, the rods in dim light and black and white vision. The human eye contains one fovea, the depression in the retina in charge of sharp central vision. The fovea is dominated by cones, the peripheral retina by rods. While you are reading this print, you are using your central vision; if someone walks into the room, you will be aware of this by the stimulation of your peripheral vision. The most accurate information is provided by the fovea, which although represents less than 2° of visual angle, is connected to 10% of the axons of the optic nerve.

Since there are 100 times the number of retinal receptors as there are nerve fibers in the optic nerve, a large amount of signal processing must be performed in the retina. Figure 1.7 describes the process by which images are compressed to fit the optic nerve capacity. The bipolar and ganglion cells perform "center surround processing" which are "on" and "off" centers. "On" centers are positively weighted in the center and negatively weighted around the center. "Off" centers are the opposite. They function similar to a mathematical algorithm in enhancing the edges of an image.

Figure 1.8 details the pathway by which the encoded image is sent via the axons of the ganglion cells through the nerve and optic chiasm to the lateral geniculate nucleus (LGN). The output of the LGN is transmitted to the visual cortex of the brain.

Fig. 1.7 Examples of the complexity of retinal organization

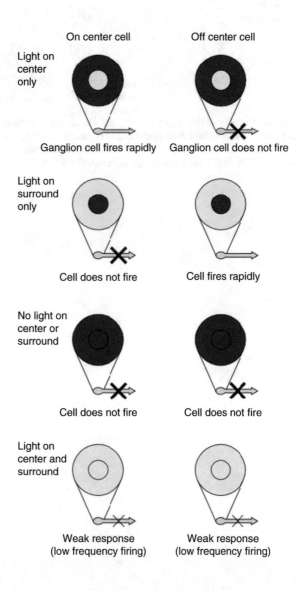

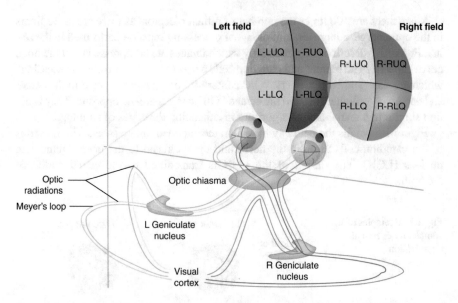

Fig. 1.8 Pathway of the encoded image sent via the axons of the ganglion cells through the nerve and optic chiasm to the lateral geniculate nucleus (LGN) of the thalamus. *L/R-LUQ* left/right eye-left upper quadrant, *L/R-LLQ* left/right eye-left lower quadrant, *L/R-RUQ* left/right eye-right upper quadrant, *L/R-RLQ* left/right eye-right lower quadrant

Chapter 2
Light Scattering

Light is a type of electromagnetic energy emitted by sources, propagated through space, and absorbed and reflected by matter. In 1801, Thomas Young developed the wave model of light. When a light wave is absorbed, the wave function collapses. The light is called a photon and represents a quantum of light. Light exhibits a wave-particle duality.

When light travels, there is an electric and a magnetic field and both rapidly oscillate at approximately 10^{14} cycles/s around zero. When a light beam hits a particle, the electric field of the light beam exerts an oscillating force on the nuclei and the electrons of the particle. While the heavier nuclei remain essentially unaffected, the lighter electrons undergo an oscillating acceleration radiating electromagnetic fields into space. The light wave energy accelerates electrons, and this energy is transferred to the particle such that light travels in all directions. The incident beam loses power. An observer can see the scattered light. If there was no scattering, to the observer the light beam would appear to be invisible. The power of the scattering medium is expressed as turbidity as it attenuates the passing light. This may be expressed as:

$$-dI = \tau I \, dz \qquad (2.1)$$

where:

z = light beam moving in a particular direction
I = light intensity at a particular position
$-dI$ = light intensity lost
τ = constant dependent on number of scattering particles, size, and polarizability or electron density in cm^{-1}

J. N. Weiss, *Dynamic Light Scattering Spectroscopy of the Human Eye*, https://doi.org/10.1007/978-3-031-06624-5_2

Fig. 2.1 Illustration of
Eq. (2.1)

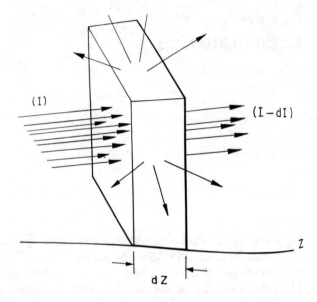

This equation applies to a thin portion of the scattering medium. Integrating Eq.
(2.1) describes the effect along the entire length of the medium (Fig. 2.1).

$$\frac{I}{I_o} = e^{-rz} \tag{2.2}$$

where:

I_o = intensity of primary beam at z = zero
I = intensity of primary beam after traversing distance z
e = natural base of logarithms

Using the normal human cornea as an example, there is an approximately 10%
loss of the primary or incident light beam traversing the cornea. If we assume the
normal corneal thickness, $z = 0.05$ cm, then $I/I_o \cong 0.90$ from Eq. (2.2). Turbidity
characterizes the quality of transparency of a scattering medium. It is apparent that
the degree of turbidity is related to the microscopic tissue structure.

How does turbidity relate to particle density? Particle shape and size will affect
its ability to scatter light. There is also a dependency of particle size as related to the
wavelength of incident light. If we assume that each particle is an independent scat-
terer, then:

$$dI = n\alpha I \, dz \tag{2.3}$$

where:

I = incident light intensity (ergs/s cm^2)
α = proportionality coefficient (light scattering effectiveness)

dz = distance traveled by light
n = number of scattering particles/unit volume

Integrating Eq. (2.3):

$$\tau = n\alpha$$

τ = constant dependent on number of scattering particles, size, and polarizability or electron density in cm^{-1} (turbidity)
n = number of scattering particles/unit volume
α = proportionality coefficient (light scattering effectiveness)

Conceptually, the turbidity increases in proportion to the density. However, this assumes independent scattering, which, in the case of the corneal collagen fibers, would cause an opaque cornea. Maurice demonstrated that the tight collagen packing within the normal, clear cornea, confirms that the fibers do not independently scatter light. If each collagen fiber is perfectly arranged, then we can calculate the relative phases and intensity of each scattered wave fields and if the distance between collagen fibers is less than the light wavelength, then the light scattered intensity is essentially zero.

Interestingly, it has been demonstrated that perfect arrangement is unnecessary. Only a limited amount of correlation is necessary to produce transparency. The uniform density of scatterers is necessary for transparency. Like the cornea, the lens of the eye consists of densely packed and uniform lens proteins and is transparent. Unlike the cornea, the lens index of refraction changes according to the anatomical location within the lens. The refraction results from scattering caused by the constructive interference of the scattered light.

Light scattering results from changes in density. The random fluctuation in density is the sum of many sinusoidal waves, also called Fourier components. When a density fluctuation causes light scattering only Fourier components with wavelengths greater than one half the wavelength of light cause the scattering.

The collagen fibers are much larger in the sclera than the cornea. The collagen diameters and fiber spacing are comparable to the wavelength of light resulting in extensive light scattering, turbidity, and an opaque sclera.

The retina exhibits a semi-regular cell arrangement packed together within small distances as compared to the light wavelength resulting in retinal transparency.

Summary of Light Scattering in the Eye

Cornea

The normal cornea accounts for 10% light scattering which is why we can study it with a slit lamp biomicroscope. We cannot visualize the corneal epithelium where the cells are held tightly together with minimal intercellular spacing. The refractive index is essentially stable so the cells appear transparent.

Lens

The normal lens absorbs visible blue light and has a slight yellow color which deepens with age. Three percent of the incident light is back scattered (Figs. 2.2 and 2.3).

Fig. 2.2 Lens of the eye

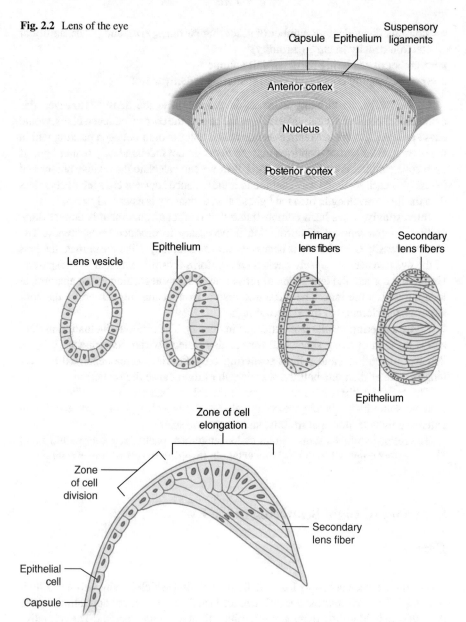

Fig. 2.3 Development of the lens

Vitreous

The vitreous body consists of hyaluronic acid molecules and collagen fibrils which are approximately 100 Å in diameter, much smaller than the normal corneal collagen fibers. Only approximately 0.1% of incident light is scattered.

Retina

The slight changes in refractive indices are small in comparison to the wavelength of light which is why the retina is transparent. The fundus is visible due to the reflection from the retinal pigment epithelium and choroid.

In order to quantify the retina light scattering, Rogers constructed a light scattering goniometer using a tunable supercontinuum laser which illuminated a 50 μm spot on an in vitro squirrel retina. His findings, below (Fig. 2.4), confirmed that the scattering coefficient was much greater in the choroid and sclera than the retina. As expected, scattering decreased with wavelength. Only the retinal pigment epithelium and choroid display absorption. Anisotropy is higher in the retina than the other structures.

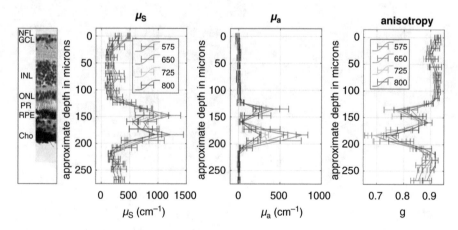

Fig. 2.4 Light scattering goniometer

Chapter 3
Dynamic Light Scattering (DLS) Spectroscopy

Dynamic Light Scattering (DLS) Spectroscopy, also known as Photon Correlation Spectroscopy (PCS), Quasielastic Light Scattering (QLS) Spectroscopy, or Laser Light Scattering (LLS) Spectroscopy measures the thermal random movement (Brownian Motion) of particles by analyzing the temporal fluctuations in scattered light intensity. The random motion of proteins causes local concentration changes which affects the intensity of scattered light. The scattered light intensity $I(t)$ is compared to the scattered light intensity at a later time, τ, measured as a time correlation $I(t + \tau)$: $< I(t)I(t + \tau)>$ where $<>$ is averaging over beginning time t. Scattered waves interference in the far field region generates a net scattered light intensity $I(t)$, which displays stochastic fluctuations depending on whether the interference is constructive or destructive due to the random motion undergone by suspended particles. DLS assumes that each detected photon has been scattered once (Fig. 3.1).

There is a high correlation with short time delays; the signals are unchanged because the particles do not have a chance to move. With a longer time delay, the correlation will decay exponentially. A monodisperse sample will exhibit a single exponential decay.

$$g(q;\tau) = \exp(-\Gamma\tau)$$

where Γ = the decay rate. The translational diffusion coefficient D_t may be derived at a single angle or at a range of angles depending on the wave vector q.

$$\Gamma = q^2 D_t$$

J. N. Weiss, *Dynamic Light Scattering Spectroscopy of the Human Eye*, https://doi.org/10.1007/978-3-031-06624-5_3

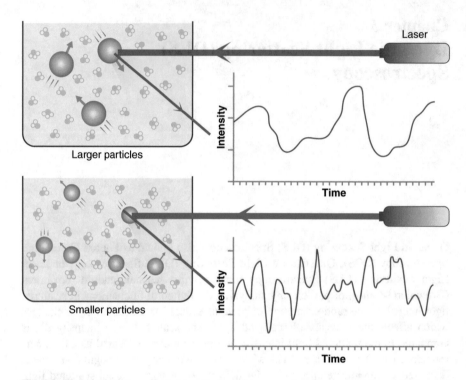

Fig. 3.1 Hypothetical dynamic light scattering of two samples: Larger particles at the top and smaller particles at the bottom

with

$$q = \frac{4\pi n0}{\lambda} \sin\left(\frac{\theta}{Q}\right)$$

where:

λ is the incident laser wavelength
n_0 is the sample's refractive index
θ is angle at which the detector is located with respect to the sample

Small spherical particles do not demonstrate angular dependence or anisotropy. Non-spherical particles demonstrate angular dependence and anisotropy.

An optimum angle of detection θ exists for each particle size. This is important in a polydisperse sample with an unknown particle size distribution. The autocorrelation function is a sum of the exponential decays corresponding to each of the species in the population.

Analysis

Cumulant Method

The cumulant method calculates the exponentials and system variance.

$$g(q;\tau) = \exp\left(-\Gamma\left(\tau - \frac{\mu_2}{2!}\tau^2 + \frac{\mu_3}{3!}\tau^3 + \cdots\right)\right)$$

where:

Γ is the average decay rate
μ_2/Γ^2 is the second order polydispersity index (variance)

The cumulant method is less affected by experimental noise.

Simply explained, a least-squares fit is made of a polynomial in *t* to the logarithm of $C(t)$, after the baseline is subtracted. *D* is the coefficient of the linear term which approximates the average particle diffusivity. An approximate particle diameter may be obtained by utilizing the Stokes-Einstein equation.

A digital autocorrelator obtains $C(t)$ simultaneously resulting in a smooth function. With uniform particles and baseline subtraction, there is a single decaying exponential.

$$C(t) = A \cdot e^{-2DK^2 t}$$

$$K = (4\pi\eta / \lambda)\sin\theta / 2)$$

where:

n = index of refraction of solvent

One obtains *D* from the decay constant. R_h, the hydrodynamic radius of the particles, is obtained by the Stokes-Einstein equation.

$$R_h = kT / 6\pi\eta D$$

where:

k = Boltzmann's constant
T = absolute temperature
η = shear viscosity of the solvent

The cumulant analysis method is simple to use. The most accurate results are achieved when applied to unimodal scattering particles with a relatively narrow size distribution. It can also provide information regarding the polydispersity of the macromolecular distribution.

The problems with this method are that it is unable to distinguish between a bimodal and a broad continuous distribution using a single sample time. Also, if there is a significant percentage of larger or aggregated particles, they will act as strong scatters and may disproportionately weight the correlation function. In this case, the diffusion coefficient will reflect the motion of the larger scatters without reflecting concentrations relative to the smaller scatterers.

CONTIN Algorithm

CONTIN uses an inverse Laplace transform to analyze the autocorrelation. It is best utilized for multimodal, heterodisperse, and polydisperse systems. The resolution for separating two different particle populations is approximately a factor of 5 or greater. The difference in relative intensities between two different populations should be less than $1:10^{-5}$.

Further Reading

1. Berne BJ, Pecora R. Dynamic light scattering. Garden City, NY: Courier Dover Publications; 2000. ISBN 0-486-41155-9
2. Chu B. Laser light scattering. Annu Rev Phys Chem. 1970;21(1):145–74. Bibcode:1970ARPC...21..145C. https://doi.org/10.1146/annurev.pc.21.100170.001045.
3. Pecora R. Doppler shifts in light scattering from pure liquids and polymer solutions. J Chem Phys. 1964;40(6):1604. Bibcode:1964JChPh..40.1604P. https://doi.org/10.1063/1.1725368.
4. Goodman J. Some fundamental properties of speckle. J Opt Soc Am. 1976;66(11):1145–50. Bibcode:1976JOSA...66.1145G. https://doi.org/10.1364/josa.66.001145.
5. Schaetzel K. Suppression of multiple-scattering by photon cross-correlation techniques. J Mod Opt. 1991;38:1849. Bibcode:1990JPCM....2..393S. https://doi.org/10.1088/0953-898 4/2/S/062.
6. Urban C, Schurtenberger P. Characterization of turbid colloidal suspensions using light scattering techniques combined with cross-correlation methods. J Colloid Interface Sci. 1998;207(1):150–8. Bibcode:1998JCIS..207..150U. https://doi.org/10.1006/jcis.1998.5769.
7. Block I, Scheffold F. Modulated 3D cross-correlation light scattering: improving turbid sample characterization. Rev Sci Instrum. 2010;81(12):123107. arXiv:1008.0615. Bibcode:2010RScI...8113107B. https://doi.org/10.1063/1.3518961.
8. Pusey PN. Suppression of multiple scattering by photon cross-correlation techniques. Curr Opin Colloid Interface Sci. 1999;4(3):177–85. https://doi.org/10.1016/S1359-0294(99)00036-9.
9. Gohy J-F, Varshney SK, Jérôme R. Water-soluble complexes formed by poly(2-vinylpyridinium)-block-poly(ethylene oxide) and poly(sodium methacrylate)-block-poly(ethylene oxide) copolymers. Macromolecules. 2001;34(10):3361. Bibcode:2001MaMol..34.3361G. https://doi.org/10.1021/ma0020483.
10. Koppel DE. Analysis of macromolecular polydispersity in intensity correlation spectroscopy: the method of cumulants. J Chem Phys. 1972;57(11):4814–20. Bibcode:1972JChPh..57.4814K. https://doi.org/10.1063/1.1678153.

11. Frisken BJ. Revisiting the method of cumulants for the analysis of dynamic light-scattering data. Appl Opt. 2001;40(24):4087–91. Bibcode:2001ApOpt..40.4087F. https://doi.org/10.1364/AO.40.004087.

12. Hassan PA, Kulshreshtha SK. Modification to the cumulant analysis of polydispersity in quasi-elastic light scattering data. J Colloid Interface Sci. 2006;300(2):744–8. Bibcode:2006JCIS ..300..744H. ISSN 0021-9797. https://doi.org/10.1016/j.jcis.2006.04.013.

13. Chu B. Laser light scattering: basic principles and practice. Academic, Boston, MA; 1992. ISBN 978-0-12-174551-6

14. Provencher S. CONTIN: a general purpose constrained regularization program for inverting noisy linear algebraic and integral equations. Comput Phys Commun. 1982;27(3):229–42. Bibcode:1982CoPhC..27..229P. https://doi.org/10.1016/0010-4655(82)90174-6.

15. Provencher SW. A constrained regularization method for inverting data represented by linear algebraic or integral equations. Comput Phys Commun. 1982;27(3):213–27. Bibcode:1982CoPhC..27..213P. https://doi.org/10.1016/0010-4655(82)90173-4.

16. Aragón SR, Pecora R. Theory of dynamic light scattering from polydisperse systems. J Chem Phys. 1976;64(6):2395. Bibcode:1976JChPh..64.2395A. https://doi.org/10.1063/1.432528.

17. Rodríguez-Fernández J, Pérez-Juste J, Liz-Marzán LM, Lang PR. Dynamic light scattering of short Au rods with low aspect ratios. J Phys Chem. 2007;111(13):5020–5. https://doi.org/10.1021/jp067049x.

18. Velu SKP, Yan M, Tseng K-P, Wong K-T, Bassani DM, Terech P. Spontaneous formation of artificial vesicles in organic media through hydrogen-bonding interactions. Macromolecules. 2013;46(4):1591–8. Bibcode:2013MaMol..46.1591V. https://doi.org/10.1021/ma302595g.

19. Jena SS, Joshi HM, Sabareesh KPV, Tata BVR, Rao TS. Dynamics of Deinococcus radiodurans under controlled growth conditions. Biophys J. 2006;91(7):2699–707. Bibcode:2006BpJ....91.2699J. https://doi.org/10.1529/biophysj.106.086520.

20. Sabareesh KPV, Jena SS, Tata BVR. Dynamic light scattering studies on photo polymerized and chemically cross-linked polyacrylamide hydrogels. AIP Conf Proc. 2006;832(1):307–10. Bibcode:2006AIPC..832..307S. ISSN 0094-243X. https://doi.org/10.1063/1.2204513.

Chapter 4
Animal Experiments

The first in vivo study of DLS was performed by Nishio, Weiss, Tanaka, et al. at M.I.T. in 1984. In this experiment, 8 New Zealand White rabbits received 2000 rads of X-irradiation (85 kVp, 5 mA) to one eye at 5 weeks of age. Matsuda, Giblin, and Reddy, in 1981, previously demonstrated that the X-irradiated lens develop posterior subcapsular opacification 3 weeks after irradiation and a mature cataract 5–6 weeks later.

A DLS system was used to perform measurements from eight irradiated and four non-irradiated control rabbits. Two irradiated rabbits were subsequently euthanized and in vitro measurements were performed. Only one eye of the rabbits was irradiated, the other eye was used as a control.

At each age, the correlation function of the lens nucleus decayed more slowly than the cortex in the normal, non-radiated rabbit with clear lenses. Older rabbits demonstrated a much slower correlation time than the younger rabbits. There was a significant decrease in correlation time as the rabbit aged from 6 to 12 weeks.

A dramatic change was observed in the correlation function of the nuclear region even 2.5 weeks after irradiation with a clear lens. The change was confirmed by both non-radiated rabbit and the opposite non-irradiated eye of the irradiated rabbit.

There was a change in the average correlation times as a function of position with the proteins at the posterior pole of the lens demonstrating a marked change in diffusivity consistent with the appearance of a posterior subcapsular cataract. The correlation time at the normal lens nucleus was larger than that found in the X-irradiated lens.

The paper showed that the in vivo measurement of lens proteins can detect cataractous changes prior to visible changes in lens turbidity (Figs. 4.1, 4.2, 4.3, 4.4, 4.5, 4.6, 4.7, and 4.8).

© The Author(s), under exclusive license to Springer Nature Switzerland AG 2022
J. N. Weiss, *Dynamic Light Scattering Spectroscopy of the Human Eye*, https://doi.org/10.1007/978-3-031-06624-5_4

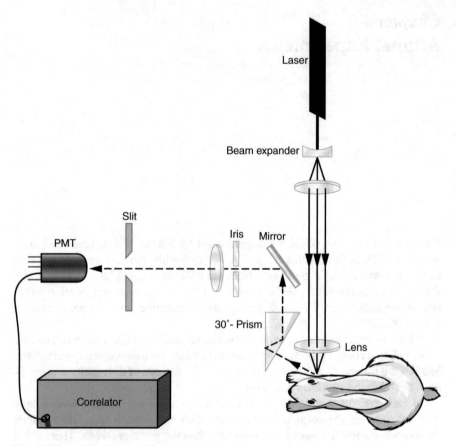

Fig. 4.1 Schematic of optical elements of DLS device

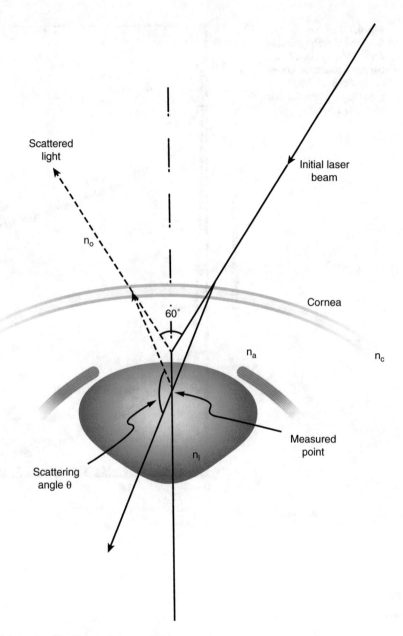

Fig. 4.2 Schematic of incident and scattered light

Fig. 4.3 Normal
8-week-old rabbit intensity
correlation function. Upper
curve = lens center. Lower
curve = anterior lens
periphery near optical axis.
(J. Weiss 12/4/83)

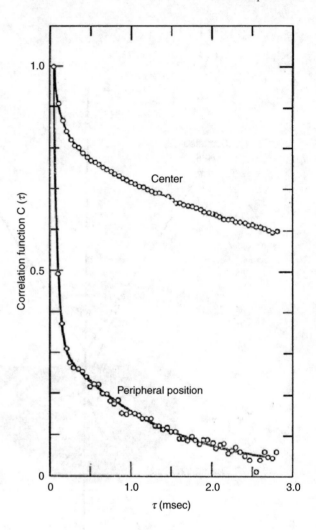

Fig. 4.4 Intensity
correlation function at
same locations taken from
a 12-week-old rabbit.
(J. Weiss 12/4/83)

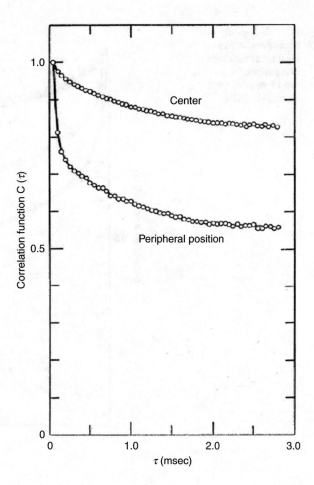

Fig. 4.5 Intensity correlation function obtained at the center of lens nucleus for 6, 8, 12, and 13-week-old non-irradiated rabbits

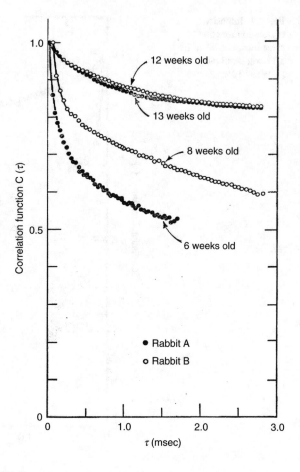

Fig. 4.6 Mean correlation time, τ, and mean diffusion coefficient, D, as function of position (non-irradiated rabbits). 8 weeks (---), 9 weeks (-·-·), 10 weeks (--), 12 weeks (····), 13 weeks (////). 1 Unit on x axis = 0.635 mm

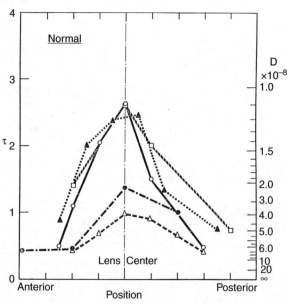

Fig. 4.7 Intensity
correlation function on
irradiated 7.5-week-old
rabbit, 2.5 weeks
post-irradiation. Top curve
from non-irradiated control
eye (left). Bottom curve
from irradiated right eye

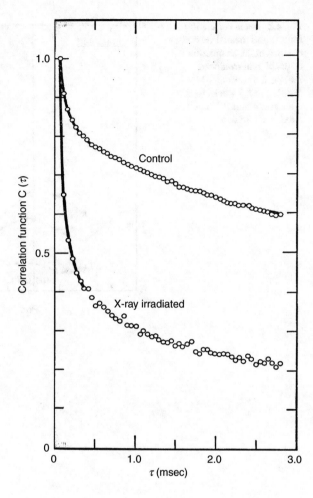

Fig. 4.8 Mean correlation
time, τ, and mean diffusion
coefficient, D, as function
of position in irradiated
rabbits. 2.5 weeks (---),
5 weeks (--), 7 weeks (....)
after irradiation. 1 Unit on
x axis = 0.635 mm

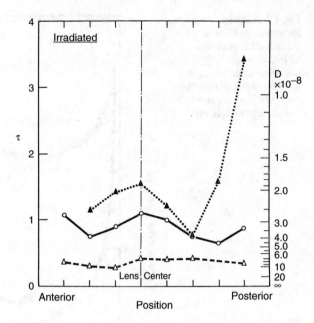

Chapter 5
Human Studies

The first DLS trial in humans was reported by Weiss and Rand, et al. in 1983. A significant correlation was found between the diffusion coefficient and patient age ($P < 0.05$). The age-adjusted mean diffusion coefficient for nondiabetics (4.60 ± 0.29; mean $\pm$ SEM) was significantly higher compared to diabetics without retinopathy (3.59 ± 0.41; $P = 0.0473$), diabetics with background or pre-proliferative retinopathy (2.73 ± 0.27; $P = 0.0001$), or to diabetics with pre-proliferative or proliferative retinopathy receiving laser photocoagulation within 1 year of measurement (3.02 ± 0.37; $P = 0.0012$). Diabetics with laser treatment more than 1 year prior to measurement (3.96 ± 0.51) did not differ significantly from nondiabetics.

The lens proteins are a polydisperse collection of scatterers with correlations from 1 µs to 1 ms sample times (Figs. 5.1, 5.2, 5.3, 5.4, and 5.5).

Bursell, Baker, Weiss, et al. performed DLS measurements on 393 diabetic patients and 38 nondiabetic patients attending the Joslin Diabetes Center Eye Unit. In order to evaluate the contributions of different protein size distributions, measurements were made at 1.5 and 150 µs sample times. The previously discovered decrease in lens protein diffusion coefficient with age was confirmed.

Age-adjusted analysis of covariance demonstrated that clinically observable nuclear sclerosis was significantly associated with a decreased diffusion coefficient. The presence of diabetes, degree of diabetic control, duration and age of onset of diabetes, and type of diabetic therapy were all significantly related to changes in the measurements of lens proteins. The lens proteins are a polydisperse collection of scatterers with correlations from 1 µs to 1 ms sample times.

Four, 5 s measurements from the lens nucleus were taken at 1.5 and 150 µs sample times. At the 1.5 µs sample time in a young group, the diffusion coefficient ranged between 1.6×10^{-7} and 6.4×10^{-8} cm²/s. The calculated hydrodynamic radii for these proteins is from 135 to 300 Å, which is comparable to the size of alpha-crystallin.

In older subjects, the calculated hydrodynamic radii was between 300 and 7000 Å, consistent with the conversion of smaller alpha-crystallin into greater

J. N. Weiss, *Dynamic Light Scattering Spectroscopy of the Human Eye*, https://doi.org/10.1007/978-3-031-06624-5_5

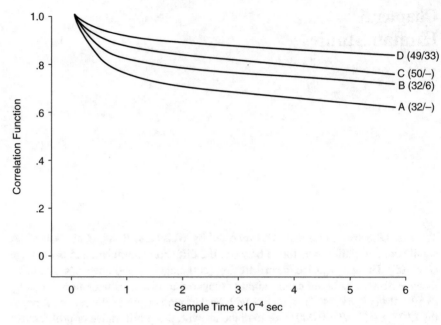

Fig. 5.1 Correlation (*r*) measured from lens nucleus. (A) 32-year-old nondiabetic, (B) 32-year-old, 6-year history of diabetes, normal retinal examination, (C) 50-year-old, nondiabetic, (D) 49-year-old, 33-year history of diabetes, normal retinal examination

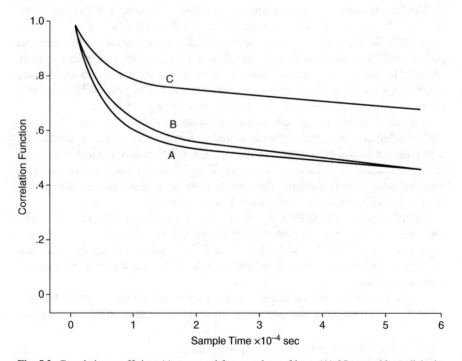

Fig. 5.2 Correlation coefficient (*r*) measured from nucleus of lens. (A) 25-year-old nondiabetic, (B) 25-year-old with 12-year history of diabetes, status post-laser photocoagulation 18 months pre-DLS measurement (OD), (C) Patient B, OS measurement (no history of laser photocoagulation)

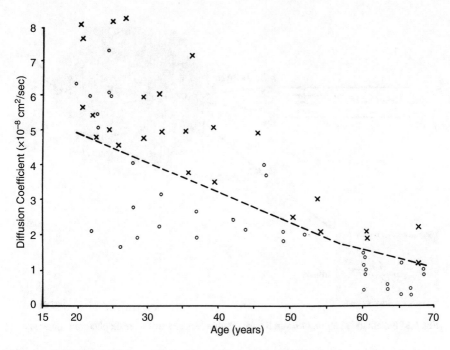

Fig. 5.3 Diffusion coefficient versus patient age. o = Diabetic patient with normal eye examination, X = Nondiabetic patient—dotted line indicates lower limit of nondiabetic data

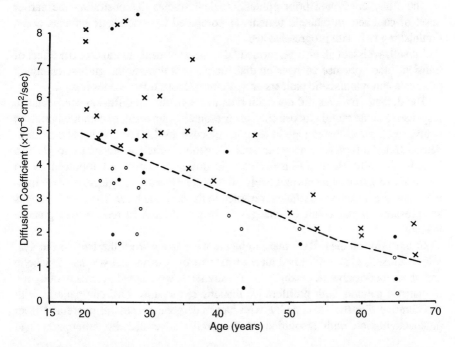

Fig. 5.4 Diffusion coefficient versus patient age for diabetic patients with pre-proliferative diabetic retinopathy, status post-laser photocoagulation • = treated eye, o = untreated eye, X = nondiabetic patients (line superimposed from Fig. 5.3)

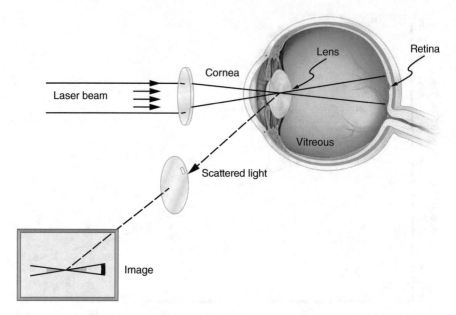

Fig. 5.5 Schematic diagram of beam focused within lens and its image on photomultiplier slit

molecular weight aggregates. The finding is consistent with biochemical studies demonstrating a decrease in alpha-crystallin monomers in the aging lens nucleus.

The study confirmed prior epidemiological studies demonstrating the earlier onset of cataracts in diabetic patients as compared to nondiabetic patients and a diminishing risk with progressive age.

Bursell, Weiss, et al. also performed DLS measurements to monitor the effect of transient blood glucose changes on diabetic patients undergoing glucose clamping protocols and nondiabetic patients undergoing glucose tolerance testing.

The diabetic patients did not exhibit an acute change in diffusion coefficient in response to acute blood glucose changes presumably the result of osmotic buffering which ameliorated the change in aqueous glucose levels. The nondiabetic patients demonstrated a biphasic change in lens diffusion coefficient secondary to glucose loading. Initially, there was a decrease in diffusion coefficient followed by an increase to a maximum approximately 30 min after peak blood glucose. Sixty minutes later, the diffusion coefficient returned to the baseline level. The noted changes are presumably the result of changes in lens hydration in response to glucose loading.

In the prior studies, DLS measurements were made from the lens of the eye. Weiss, Bursell, et al. performed measurements from the corneal stroma of diabetic and nondiabetic patients. Changes in measurements were noted as a result of aging, in diabetic patients with proliferative diabetic retinopathy. Diabetic patients with proliferative diabetic retinopathy, who had undergone successful panretinal laser photocoagulation with resolution of the proliferative diabetic retinopathy had measurements similar to nondiabetics or to diabetic patients without retinopathy, or with minimal background diabetic retinopathy.

In the 1980s, both Alcon and Allergan had programs attempting to develop a cure for cataracts. Two DLS units were constructed for these companies. Unfortunately, both companies discontinued their search for anti-cataract agents (Figs. 5.6 and 5.7).

In 2018, a new DLS machine was designed and built for the purpose of making retinal measurements (Fig. 5.8).

Weiss conducted the first study utilizing retinal DLS measurements in patients receiving intravitreal injections of either Avastin, Lucentis, or Eylea for wet age-related macular degeneration. Ten patients receiving these injections underwent DLS measurements over the course of 6 months to determine whether the measurement could predict the redevelopment of subretinal fluid in patients receiving these medications.

The study results may be summarized as follows:

1. Each patient is their own control.
2. If the right eye (OD) or left eye (OS) fundus is normal, then the measurements between the two eyes are within a few percent of each other.
3. DLS measurements are reproducible over time.

Fig. 5.6 Original DLS machine

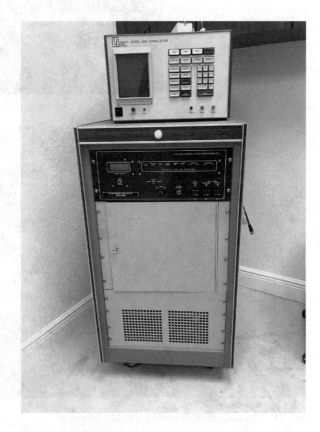

Fig. 5.7 Sample data from
original DLS machine

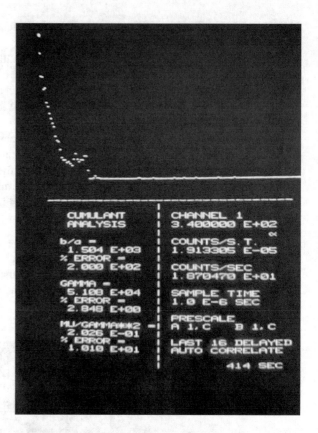

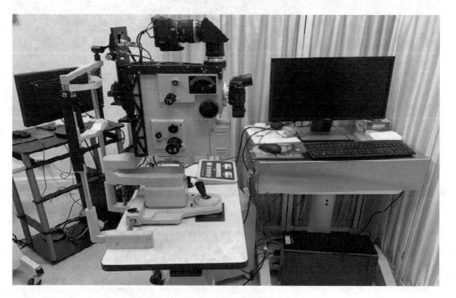

Fig. 5.8 New dynamic light scattering (DLS) device

4. DLS measurements decrease in eyes requiring the anti-VEGF medication and anticipates or predicts the development of subretinal fluid.
5. The DLS measurement increases in those patients with successful response to injections with a decrease in subretinal fluid and decreases in those patients requiring additional injections.
6. DLS measurements anticipate OCT results.
7. DLS measurements more accurately mirror visual acuity than does OCT.
8. Increased DLS measurements and increased visual acuity is observed, even if the OCT measurement is unchanged.
9. Eyes that have received Avastin or Lucentis, even if stable, have a lower DLS measurement than the fellow, untreated eye. The observed lower DLS measurement is similar to that obtained in patients diagnosed with geographic atrophy.
10. Eyes that received Eylea did not exhibit the significant decrease in DLS measurements seen in patients receiving either Avastin or Lucentis.

In another study, DLS measurements were performed in a patient with a history of nonarteritic ischemic optic neuropathy (NAION) that underwent stem cell treatment within the IRB-approved Stem Cell Ophthalmology Treatment Study (SCOTS). An increase in the DLS measurement was seen paralleling the improvement in visual acuity and visual field, despite an absence of change in the fundus and OCT examinations (Fig. 5.9).

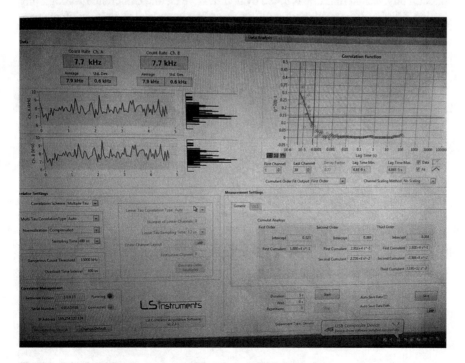

Fig. 5.9 Sample DLS measurement utilizing the new DLS device

At the present time, we have undertaken a study utilizing DLS equipment to detect Alzheimer's disease. The study protocol and informed consent are included.

Alzheimer's Disease is a progressive, degenerative brain disorder leading to death. Early-onset Alzheimer's disease (ages 30–65) is strongly related to hereditary and genetics. Late-onset Alzheimer's (age 65 and older) is the leading cause of dementia, affected more than five million Americans. While associated with advancing age, there is no evidence that the disease is caused by the aging process. While particular genes may increase susceptibility to late-onset Alzheimer's, researchers are studying the effect of genetic, environmental, dietary, infectious agents, and metabolic abnormalities that may lead to the diseases' development.

Unfortunately, there is no clinical test to diagnose this condition. Posthumously, neuritic plaques composed of amyloid protein and/or neurofibrillary tangles of tau protein are found. The average life expectancy following diagnosis is 5–10 years. There is no successful treatment, drugs may improve symptoms in some cases.

In the last decade, more than 500 drug studies have failed to find a treatment for this condition. In the absence of a definitive quantitative endpoint, most studies have been terminated after 2 years, yet it would take more than 5 years to determine a meaningful effect.

The eye is the only place in the body where an artery, vein, and nerve can be directly visualized. The nerve fiber layer of the retina is an outgrowth of the brain. Recent research has determined that the retina is affected by Alzheimer's disease. Specifically, retinal thinning is noted by noninvasive Ocular Coherence Tomography testing. Obviously, a much earlier molecular effect must lead to an imaging change.

Chapter 6
Neurologic Diseases: Protocol

Dynamic Light Scattering Ocular Measurement of Patients with Dementia

Introduction

Type of Research

This is a human clinical study making a noninvasive measurement from a patient's eye to determine whether there is a quantitative difference in measurement between patients with and without the diagnosis of dementia.

This research is not federally funded nor subject to federal oversight. There is no HDE involved.

Purpose and Objective of the Study

The purpose of the study is to determine whether dynamic light scattering spectroscopy, also known as laser light scattering spectroscopy, or photon correlation spectroscopy, a noninvasive quantitative technique, has utility in the diagnosis of dementia. The objective is to determine which types of dementia and at what stages they may be most effectively detected.

Background of the Study

Study Rationale

Dementia is a common cause of morbidity and mortality. It is caused by physical changes in the brain that causes the loss of mental abilities and memory that affect the activities of daily living. The types of dementia include: Alzheimer's disease,

© The Author(s), under exclusive license to Springer Nature
Switzerland AG 2022
J. N. Weiss, *Dynamic Light Scattering Spectroscopy of the Human Eye*,
https://doi.org/10.1007/978-3-031-06624-5_6

Vascular dementia, Dementia with Lewy bodies, Mixed dementia, Parkinson's disease, Frontotemporal dementia, Creutzfeldt-Jakob disease, Normal pressure hydrocephalus, Huntington's disease, Wernicke-Korsakoff Syndrome, etc.

Alzheimer's disease is a slowly progressive brain disease beginning prior to the appearance of symptoms and accounts for approximately 60–80% of dementia cases. Definitive diagnosis is made posthumously with the discovery of protein fragment beta-amyloid plaques and twisted strands of the protein tau (tangles) with nerve cell damage and death.

Vascular dementia, previously known as post-stroke or multi-infarct dementia is solely diagnosed in approximately 10% of dementia cases. The development of Lewy bodies in the cerebral cortex can cause dementia. The type of aggregate pattern may be indicative of Dementia with Lewy bodies or of Parkinson's disease.

Abnormalities of more than one dementia cause may occur simultaneously in the brain causing a mixed dementia. In Parkinson's disease, the alpha-synuclein clumps generally occur in a deep area of the brain called the substantia nigra and are thought to affect the production of dopamine.

In Normal Pressure Hydrocephalus, an abnormal increase of fluid in the brain leads to dementia. This may sometimes be corrected by the placement of a shunt in the brain to drain the excess fluid. There are no definite distinguishing microscopic abnormalities seen in all cases of frontotemporal dementia.

Creutzfeldt-Jakob disease (mad-cow disease) is caused by an infection with a prion. Huntington's disease is caused by a defective gene on chromosome 4. Vitamin B-1 deficiency (thiamine), generally caused by alcoholism, is the cause of Wernicke-Korsakoff syndrome.

In the absence of dementia etiology, as seen in Creutzfeldt-Jakob disease, Normal Pressure Hydrocephalus, Huntington's disease, Wernicke-Korsakoff syndrome, the true diagnosis is generally made pathologically, after the patient has expired.

During the last 15 years, there have been more than 500 clinical trials of therapeutic agents for Alzheimer's disease registered with the National Institute of Health website, clinicaltrials.gov. For those trials with reported results, the failure rate has been almost 100%. Though most trials typically last 1.5–3 years, it has been estimated that, depending on the efficacy of the therapeutic intervention, study duration would need to be 5–10 years in duration to detect an effect.

Therefore, what is needed is a sensitive, quantitative, technique that can detect the beginnings or early onset of these conditions before the development of symptoms.

The retina is visible within the eye and is composed of nine histologic layers. The nerve fiber layer of the retina is an extension of the brain. The early detection of neurologic damage at the microscopic level when it is still potentially reversible is a prerequisite for the development of potential cures. The early detection of the effectiveness of treatment allows for better and more effective treatments.

It has been demonstrated that patients with Alzheimer's disease have thinning of the retinal nerve fiber layer and retinal ganglion cell layer by ocular coherence tomography (OCT) images and measurements taken through the macula and peripapillary areas. This was consistent with histopathologic data. Inner retina thinning has been correlated with disease severity. This may be related to the presence of amyloid-beta within the retina.

Inner retinal thinning has been found in other neurodegenerative diseases including multiple sclerosis, amyotrophic lateral sclerosis, dementia with Lewy bodies, and multiple system atrophy.

As compared to the inner retinal thinning seen in Alzheimer's disease, thinning of the photoreceptor or outer retina thinning has been found in frontotemporal degeneration. Approximately 30% of patients initially diagnosed with frontotemporal degeneration are subsequently diagnosed with Alzheimer's disease at autopsy.

Dynamic Light Scattering (DLS) measures the scattered light intensity fluctuations resulting from thermal random motion (Brownian motion). It has been used to predict the development of cataracts in rabbits and detect the development of cataract formation and of diabetes mellitus in humans. The results demonstrated the utility of DLS to noninvasively quantitate subtle changes at the molecular level.

A proof-of-concept instrument for making retinal measurements was developed. The system provides optical power below the maximal permissible exposure recommended by the ANSI Z136.1 (2014) standard. The minimal amount of light necessary to make a 5 s measurement is used. The detection system is interfaced with a standard clinical fundus camera.

The scattered light is analyzed by a digital autocorrelator with an extended delay option for baseline determination. The intensity fluctuations are averaged over 5 s and the cumulant analysis method used to analyze the resulting autocorrelation function. Diffusion coefficient, decay times, and polydispersity factors, as a function of the sample time, are also calculated.

Seventeen patients were tested using this device and no significant difference was seen between the left and the right eye in patients with normal eye examinations. In addition, the results, taken over a 6-month time span were not significantly different, demonstrating a reproducibility and consistency of measurement.

A 69-year-old man with a 16-month history of acute visual loss of the left eye (OS) to Counting Fingers (CF) at 6′, diagnosed with non-arteritic ischemic optic neuropathy (NAION), acutely lost vision in his right eye (OD) 8 months later to CF at 3′, also secondary to NAION. The patient underwent retinal stem cell surgery according to the IRB-approved SCOTS II protocol.

The DLS device quantitatively detected and predicted visual improvement following stem cell surgery in the absence of changes in imaging as observed by standard ophthalmologic testing. In addition, though early baseline measurements were similar, the greater visual improvement of the patient's left eye as compared to the right eye was also detected by the DLS device.

The ability to quantitatively and objectively detect molecular changes, before they become observable by standard imaging techniques allows the early detection and monitoring of patients with conditions affecting the retina, such as dementia.

Participant Selection

1. Inclusion and Exclusion Criteria

    Inclusion:

    To be eligible for the study patients must:

    > Have documented diagnosis of dementia or no neurologic condition of cerebral origin.
    > Have no ophthalmic history of pathology, except for refractive error or cataract.
    > Be over the age of 18.
    > Be medically stable.

    Restrictions:

    > All patients must be capable of an adequate ophthalmic evaluation and testing. This includes the ability to cooperate with the exam, sufficiently clear media (cornea, lens, vitreous) and sufficient pupillary dilation.
    > Patients must be capable of providing informed consent.
    > Patients who are not medically stable or who may be at significant risk to their health will not be eligible.
    > Women of child-bearing age must not be pregnant at the time of examination.

2. Gender—no restrictions. Women of child-bearing age are eligible but must not be pregnant at the time of treatment.
3. Racial/Ethnic origin—no restrictions.
4. Vulnerable populations—no vulnerable populations will be eligible.
5. Age—no patients under the age of 18 are to be enrolled. For those 18 years and older there will be no age restrictions.
6. Total number of participants to be enrolled: 50.

    > 25 patients diagnosed with dementia
    > 25 age-matched patients without cerebral pathology

Study Design/Method/Procedures

Summary of Research Design

This is an office-based study. Patients referred by Dr. _____ for study inclusion will be interviewed. An ophthalmic history will be taken. If the patient is eligible for study participation, they will under pharmacologic dilation of one eye. Standard ophthalmic drops used for mydriasis will be utilized. After approximately

10–15 min, a DLS measurement will be performed. It is estimated that the two tests will take 5 min to complete. The patient will be instructed that the dilation will wear off in approximately 1–2 h.

Performance of Measurements

Dynamic Light Scattering (DLS) Device – The patient fixates with their undilated eye at an external light. The standard, commercially available fundus camera is focused on the retina. The DLS light is parfocal with the fundus camera. The DLS operator (Dr. Weiss) presses a button and a 5 s duration measurement is made.

General Side Effects

The procedure includes the administration of standard ophthalmic medications to dilate the pupil. There is a very small chance that this may lead to an angle closure glaucoma. This is unlikely and has not been seen in Dr. Weiss' more than 30-year career as an ophthalmologist.

Collection and Used of Data

Patients give permission for use of their medical information, for their own care, and for any publication, presentation, or public communication about the procedure and results. In the case of non-direct patient care communication, the patient's name and contact information will be held in confidence and not released to protect privacy. However, if required by law, state, or federal agencies may be given access to the full name, data, medical records, and information. Access will be granted to the Institutional Review Board as they require for monitoring of the IRB.

Analysis of Study Results

Data will be collected and analyzed for significance. Standard statistical methodology will be used.

Storage of Data

Data will be stored in paper files and will be accessible by Dr. Weiss, his staff and associates. This will be kept in the usual manner as other medical files and for the required period of time as provided by state of Florida law.

Confidentiality of Data

All data will be maintained in a confidential manner equal to other medical data and records.

Risk/Benefit Assessment

Risk and discomforts are Minimal Risk. Pupillary dilation is a normal part of standard eye examination. The measurement light is much weaker than those lights used in a standard eye examination.

Adverse Events

Any Adverse Events (AE) or Serious Adverse Events (SAE) will be managed by Dr. Weiss at the time of the event. An Adverse Event will be defined as an event related to the procedure that has a high risk to cause permanent loss of vision or health to the patient. These will be reported to IRB with 60 days of documentation. A Serious Adverse Event will be defined as permanent loss of vision or permanent medical injury to the patient as a result of the procedure and will be reported to IRB within 45 business days of their documentation.

Benefits

Patients participating in this study will receive no direct benefits other than possibly contributing to helping other patients with dementia.

Participant Recruitment and Informed Consent

Recruiting

Recruiting will be brought to the attention of potential patients through announcements made by Dr. _____ office. Recruiting will continue until 50 patients have been enrolled. No coercion will be used. In the course of providing information about the study, it will be communicated that patients will be participating in a clinical study conducted under an IRB-approved protocol.

Length of Study

The study will begin on the date of IRB approval and continue until 50 patients are recruited for the study. It is estimated that it will take less than 1 year to complete the study.

Informed Consent/Assent

See Informed Consent Chap. 7.

Chapter 7
Neurologic Diseases: Informed Consent

Dynamic Light Scattering Ocular Measurement of Patients with Dementia

Introduction

To decide whether or not you want to have a special measurement made from your eye, the risks and possible benefits are described in this form so that you can make an informed decision. This process is known as informed consent. This consent form describes the purpose, procedures, possible benefits, and risks of the procedure. You may have a copy of this form to review at your leisure or to ask advice from others.

Dr. Weiss and his associates will answer any questions you may have about this form or about the procedure. Please read this document carefully and do not hesitate to ask anything about this information. This form may contain words that you do not understand. Please ask Dr. Weiss or his associates to explain the words or information that you do not understand. After reading (or having it read to you) the consent form, if you would like to be tested you will be asked to sign this form.

Terms of the Study

Dr. Weiss will determine if you are eligible for inclusion in the study. If you have been approved for inclusion in the study, you are being asked to participate in a clinical research study to determine if the eye measurement is related to the diagnosis of cognitive impairment.

There will be approximately 50 participants enrolled in the study at one site in the United States.

J. N. Weiss, *Dynamic Light Scattering Spectroscopy of the Human Eye*,
https://doi.org/10.1007/978-3-031-06624-5_7

Reproductive Information for Females

There is no evidence that the eye measurement will affect pregnancy.

Benefits/Outcome of Treatment

Patients participating in this study will receive no direct benefits other than possibly contributing to helping other patients with dementia.

In signing this informed consent, you acknowledge that no promise of beneficial results has been made to you, nor have any guarantees been offered, either formally or implied, that the eye measurement will be successful or be of benefit.

Description of Procedure

Traditional eye drops as used in your eye doctor's office will be used to dilate one eye. You may choose which eye you want dilated. The drops normally require approximately 10–15 min to dilate the pupil. You will be asked to look at a blinking light and a 5 s measurement will be made from the eye.

This permission also provides for access to your follow-up neurologic exams to Dr. Weiss and his associates and the ability to discuss your treatment and results freely with your health providers.

Cost

There is no cost for this procedure.

Collection and Use of Data

Patients give permission for use of their medical information for their own care and for any publication, presentation, or public communication about the procedure and results. Your name and contact information will be held in confidence and not released to protect your privacy. However, if required by law, state or federal agencies may be given access to your full name, data, medical records, and information.

Confidentiality of Records

You understand that your identity and certain information pertaining to you that is collected for this study will remain confidential. However, in order to meet the obligations of Federal law, you understand that records from this study may be subject to review by representatives of the Institutional Review Board and authorized Food and Drug Administration or other government regulatory agencies' personnel. You hereby consent to such review and disclosure.

Available Information

If you have any questions or desire further information with respect to this study, you may contact:
Jeffrey N. Weiss, MD
821 Coral Ridge Drive
Coral Springs, FL 33071

Termination

You understand that your participation in this study is voluntary, and you are under no obligation to participate. Your decision on whether to participate in the study will in no way impact upon the treatment you will receive. You may refuse to participate or may discontinue at any time during the study without penalty.

Participant Statement and Authorization

In affixing my signature, I acknowledge that I have read or had read to me this informed consent and permission form, that all my questions have been answered and that I fully understand the information it contains. I consent to the eye measurement as performed by Dr. Jeffrey Weiss and his associates.

_____

Printed Name of Patient

_____   _____
Signature of Patient   Date

_____

Name of and relationship of responsible party if patient unable to sign

_____   _____
Signature of responsible party if patient unable to sign   Date

_____
Printed name of person explaining consent

_____   _____
Signature of person explaining consent   Date

Chapter 8
Patents: Apparatus for the Detection of Diabetes and Other Abnormalities Affecting the Lens of the Eye

United States Patent	4,883,351
Weiss	November 28, 1989

Inventors:	Weiss; Jeffrey N. (Brookline, MA)
Family ID:	27023441
Appl. No.:	06/671,520
Filed:	November 15, 1984

Related U.S. Patent Documents

Application Number	Filing Date	Patent Number	Issue Date
416654	Sep 10, 1982		

Current U.S. Class:	351/221; 600/318; 600/319; 607/89; 128/897; 351/214; 606/4
Current CPC Class:	A61B 3/1173 (20130101); A61B 5/14532 (20130101); A61B 5/1455 (20130101); A61B 5/411 (20130101)
Current International Class:	A61B 3/117 (20060101); A61B 3/12 (20060101); A61B 5/00 (20060101); A61B 003/10 ()
Field of Search:	;351/210,211,214,221

© The Author(s), under exclusive license to Springer Nature
Switzerland AG 2022
J. N. Weiss, *Dynamic Light Scattering Spectroscopy of the Human Eye*,
https://doi.org/10.1007/978-3-031-06624-5_8

References Cited [Referenced by]

U.S. Patent Documents

4477159	October 1984	Mizuno et al.

Other References

Tanaka et al., Investigative Ophthalmology and Visual Science, vol. 16, pp. 135–140, Feb. 19, 1977.

Primary Examiner: Arnold; Bruce Y.
Assistant Examiner: Dzierzynski; P. M.
Attorney, Agent or Firm: Wolf, Greenfield & Sacks, P.C.

Parent Case Text

Cross-reference to Related Applications

This application is a division of my parent patent application Ser. No. 416,654, now abandoned filed Sept. 10, 1982. Continuation of the parent patent application was filed on Nov. 19, 1984, and has been given Ser. No. 672,717.

Claims

I Claim

1. In apparatus for measuring the movement of light scattering elements in the lens of an in vivo eye where the apparatus is of the type having the following:

   (a) Means for providing a beam of light.
   (b) Means for focusing the light beam on a site in the lens of the eye.
   (c) A photomultiplier.
   (d) Optical means for transmitting light back-scattered from the eye's lens to the photomultiplier.
   (e) Correlator means for providing an output that is an autocorrelation function of light intensity variations affecting the photomultiplier's output, the improvement wherein the optical means for transmitting light back-scattered

from the eye's lens to the photomultiplier is an optical fiber having a light receiving input end, and the improvement further comprises the following:

   (i) A binocular microscope for providing a stereoscopic view of the site at which the light beam is focused on the lens, the optical axis of the binocular microscope being directed at an angle to the light beam sufficient to provide depth perception.

   (ii) The optical fiber having its input end disposed to enable the binocular microscope to focus light back-scattered from the eye's lens upon the input end of the optical fiber without impairing the stereoscopic view of the site.

2. The improvement according to claim 1, wherein the input end of the optical fiber is disposed in an eyepiece of the binocular microscope.

3. The apparatus according to claim 2, wherein the means for providing a beam light is a laser, and wherein the improvement further comprises the following:

   (iii) A slit lamp for providing a beam of light in addition to the laser's beam, the slit lamp being parfocal with the laser.

Description

Field of the Invention

This invention relates to medical diagnostic and monitoring apparatus and, in particular, to apparatus for detecting and monitoring diabetes mellitus and other abnormalities affecting the lens of an eye.

Background of the Invention

Diabetes mellitus is one of the leading causes of morbidity and mortality in the United States. Although the disease, once diagnosed, can be controlled, the diabetic patient faces many complications, some of them life-threatening. For example, the average life expectancy of the diabetic patient is one-third less than that of the general population; blindness is 25 times as common, renal disease is 17 times more common, gangrene is 5 times as common, and heart disease is twice as common in diabetics as compared to the nondiabetic.

In addition, the incidence of this disease appears to be increasing—between 1936 and 1978 there was a sixfold increase in the prevalence of the disease.

It is believed by many researchers in the field that many complications suffered by diabetic patients can be minimized or avoided by early detection of the onset of the disease and proper long-term control of the patient's blood glucose.

Unfortunately, prior art detection and monitoring methods and apparatus have been unable to either accurately detect the onset of the disease at an early stage or assess the degree of control on a long-term basis. Such prior art detection methods, other than interpretation of clinical symptoms, rely on blood sugar measurements which reflect the presence of the disease. Prior art monitoring methods involve either spot blood sugar measurements or more complicated blood tests which reflect blood glucose levels that existed in the patient's body at a time 3–5 weeks prior to the time of measurement. Both prior art measurement methods require bodily invasion and the results are difficult to interpret.

Accordingly, it is an object of this invention to provide apparatus to detect the onset of diabetes mellitus prior to the appearance of clinical symptoms.

It is another object of this invention to provide apparatus for the detection of abnormalities affecting the lens of the eye.

It is still another object of this invention to provide apparatus which facilitates assessment of the effectiveness of various methods of diabetic treatment.

It is yet another object of this invention to provide apparatus which conduces to the ascertainment of the degree of control required to prevent the occurrence of diabetic complications.

It is a further object of this invention to provide an apparatus which enables the effects of systemic disease, trauma, drugs, local inflammatory conditions of the eye, and aging to be quantified by measurements taken from the lens of an in vivo eye.

Summary of the Invention

The foregoing objects are achieved and the foregoing problems are solved in one illustrative embodiment of the invention in which the diffusion coefficient of the lens of a patient's eye is measured by directing the beam from a low-power laser at the patient's lens and measuring the intensity of the back-scattered light. A number of measurements are taken of the diffusion coefficient for patients known to be normal to establish a diffusion coefficient-age relationship. The lens diffusion coefficient of an unknown patient is compared to the pre-established relationship and a significant decrease of lens diffusion coefficient over the normal diffusion coefficient-age relationship indicates a likelihood of diabetes. The amount of decrease of lens diffusion coefficient over the normal pre-established diffusion coefficient can be used to indicate the severity of the disease or monitor the progress and treatment of the disease.

More particularly, the optical system used in illustrative embodiment consists of a low-power laser and associated optics attached to a slit-lamp biomicroscope equipped with precision mechanical adjustments to focus the light beam on a site in the patient's lens. A photomultiplier is used to detect the intensity of light back-scattered from the site and a correlator is used to process the output of the photomultiplier to provide a set of numbers that can be used to calculate the diffusion coefficient.

Brief Description of the Drawings

Figure 8.1 is a perspective view of the slit-lamp biomicroscope and added equipment used to focus the light beam on a site in the patient's lens

Figure 8.2 shows an overall schematic view of the optical arrangement to irradiate a site in the patient's lens and the apparatus used to process the resulting signal.

Figure 8.3 shows a graph of lens diffusion coefficient versus patient age developed using the apparatus of the present invention which graph is useful in detecting and monitoring diabetes

Detailed Description of the Preferred Embodiment

Figure 8.1 shows the mechanical and optical arrangement for an illustrative embodiment of the inventive diabetic detection device. In particular, a suitable arrangement consists of a modification of a commercially available optical instrument known as

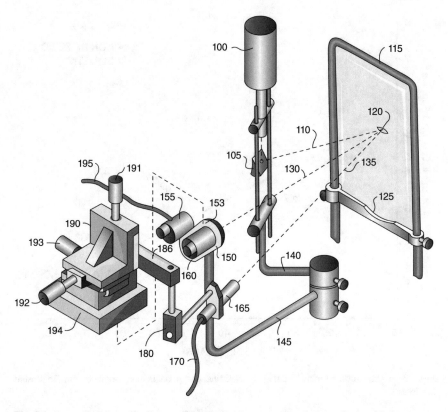

Fig. 8.1 A non-limiting embodiment of the electronic components in accordance with the present disclosure

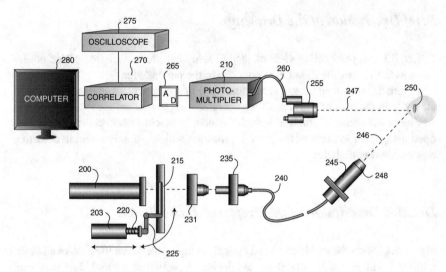

Fig. 8.2 A non-limiting attachment of the optical system to the fundus camera

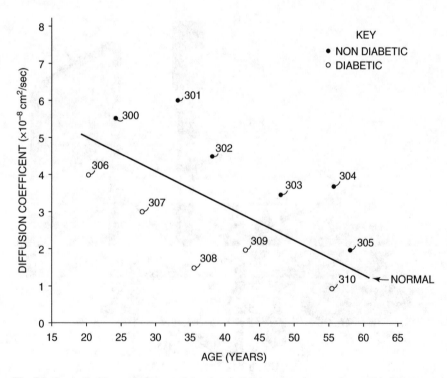

Fig. 8.3 A non-limiting embodiment of the electrical components in accordance with the present disclosure

a slit-lamp biomicroscope. This device is well-known to those skilled in the art and typically is used in ophthalmological studies of the cornea, lens, and retina of the human eye. A device suitable for use with the illustrative embodiment is manufactured by several companies and its operation and use are well-known to those skilled in the art.

Basically, a slit-lamp biomicroscope consists of a light source, a microscope, and a mechanical supporting arrangement which allows precise positioning of the light source and microscope relative to the patient to allow focusing of the light on selected sites in the patient's eye. Specifically, light produced by source 100 is reflected from mirror 105 and directed as beam 110 to the patient's eye shown schematically as eye 120. The apparatus also includes frame 115 and support 125 which position and hold the patient's head in a fixed position. Light which is reflected or scattered by the patient's cornea, lens, or retina, shown schematically as beam 130, is received by a binocular microscope arrangement 150 which has two eyepieces, 155 and 160. The lamp arrangement and microscope are supported by arms 140 and 145 from a common post, all in a well-known manner.

In accordance with the invention, the standard slit-lamp biomicroscope is modified by the addition of an *XYZ* positioning apparatus to the microscope arrangement 150. In particular, the *XYZ* position apparatus consists of commercial *XYZ* positioner 190 which can obtain precise three-dimensional movement which is controlled by three orthogonal micrometers, 191–193. Positioner 190 is mounted on plate 194 which is in turn fastened to microscope arrangement 150 by means of a threaded hole 153 which is normally found on the arrangement and used for other purposes.

Attached to the movable surface of *XYZ* positioner 190 are arms 180 and 186 which support a lens arrangement 165. As will be hereinafter further explained, lens arrangement 165 is connected via fiber optic cable 170 to a laser and used to illuminate the patient's lens via beam 135. The back-scattered light shown schematically as beam 130 is detected by a sensor located in the focal plane of eyepiece 155 and conveyed via cable 195 to a photomultiplier (not shown).

Figure 8.2 of the drawing shows a schematic diagram of the entire optical arrangement of the present invention. The apparatus consists of an irradiating portion or light source for illuminating the patient's lens and a detecting or receiving portion for receiving the back-scattered radiation.

The light source part of the apparatus consists of laser 200, two filters mounted in housing 215, microscope objective lens 231, fiber optic termination 235, fiber optic cable 240, and focusing lens arrangement 245. Laser 200 is a 5-mW helium-neon laser of conventional design which is commercially available from several companies. A laser suitable for use with the illustrative embodiment is a model U-1305P manufactured by the Newport Corporation, 18235 Mount Baldy Circle, Fountain Valley, Calif. The output of laser 200 passes through two neutral density filters, mounted in housing 215. One filter is permanently mounted in the laser beam path and reduced the power output of laser 200 to 1.5 mW. The other filter is solenoid-controlled so that it can automatically be moved out of the laser beam path during the measurement operation. When both filters are in place, they reduce the laser output power to 0.50 mW. The movable filter is used during premeasurement focusing, as will hereinafter be described, in order to reduce the patient's exposure to unnecessary laser irradiation. The movable filter is controlled by solenoid 203 which is under control of a footswitch operated by the person making the measurement. When solenoid 203 is operated, arm 220 retracts, in turn, sliding the movable filter in housing 215 by means of bell-crank 225.

After passing through one or both filters, the attenuated laser output light enters lens 231. Lens 231 is a 40× microscope objective lens which is mounted so that it focuses the laser light on the end of the optical fiber which transmits the light to the irradiating apparatus. Light passing through lens 231 falls onto an optical fiber 240 mounted in termination 235. The end of fiber 240 which enters termination 235 is attached to an XYZ positioner. The positioner is used to align the end of the optical fiber with the focusing lens to obtain maximum light transmission.

The other end of optical fiber 240 is attached to focusing lens arrangement 245. Lens arrangement 245 consists of a fiber optic holder which is slidably mounted in a lens holder tube. Lens 248 is an 18 mm focal-length converging lens which is mounted at the other end of the lens holder tube. The movable arrangement between the fiber optic holder and the lens allows small adjustments to be made between the end of the optical fiber and the lens to permit fine focusing of the laser output beam at a given position within the patient's lens.

Lens arrangement 245 is connected to the XYZ positioner attached to the slit-lamp biomicroscope as previously described and is used to focus the laser beam, 246, such that a sharp focus is achieved at the patient's lens 250. After passing through the focal point in the lens, the beam becomes sharply defocused in order to maintain a low irradiation level at the retina and prevent any possibility of injury or damage.

The detection optical system uses portions of the optical system of the slit-lamp biomicroscope. In particular, light back-scattered from the patient's lens (represented schematically as beam 247) is focused by one objective of the binocular portion of microscope 255 onto a commercially available optical fiber light guide, 260, located at the center of the focal point of the eyepiece. In the illustrative embodiment, the end termination of optical fiber light guide 260 replaces the normal left ocular of slit-lamp biomicroscope 255. The arrangement is such that the end of fiber cable 260 can be seen when looking through the left ocular to allow focusing of the back-scattered radiation on the end of the fiber cable. Scattered light received at microscope 255 is fed by fiber optic guide 260 to photomultiplier 210 which is a well-known, commercially available device. A photomultiplier suitable for use with the illustrative embodiment is a model number 9863B/350 manufactured by EMI Gencom, Inc., 80 Express Street, Plainview, N.Y. The output of photomultiplier 210 is provided to amplifier-discriminator 265 which also is a well-known device that amplifies the output pulse signals produced by the photomultiplier and selectively sends to correlator 270 only those signals which have an amplitude above a preset threshold. A suitable amplifier-discriminator for use with the illustrative embodiment is a model number AD6 manufactured by Pacific Photometric Instruments, Inc., 5675 Landregan Street, Emeryville, Calif.

The output of amplifier-discriminator 265 is, in turn, provided to a commercial photon correlation spectrometer 270 (a suitable spectrometer is a model DC64 manufactured by Langley-Ford Instruments, 85 North Whitney Street, Amherst, Mass.). Correlator 270 counts the number of pulses received from amplifier-discriminator 265 for a predetermined time interval and performs a well-known mathematical operation to obtain the correlation function. In the illustrative embodiment, a suitable time interval is 10 μs. The correlator utilizes these received counts to solve the following equation for the autocorrelation function $C_m(t)$:

$$C_m\left(t\right) = \sum_{i=1}^{i=n} p_i p_i + m$$

where

t = the length of the predetermined time interval
i = an index number whose range is one to the total number of intervals
p_i = the number of pulses occurring during the ith time interval
n = the total number of intervals
m = an integer whose range is 1–64

In accordance with the above equation, correlator 270 produces solutions or points (one for each value of m) in a time sequence, each measurement separated by the value of t. These measurements may be plotted against time to produce a curve which may then be displayed for examination on oscilloscope 275. The values of the solutions may also be provided to computer 280 for further processing to determine the diffusion coefficient. A computer suitable for use with the illustrative embodiment is a personal computer manufactured by the International Business Machines Corporation, Armonk, New York.

In particular, the diffusion coefficient (D) is also related to the correlation function $C_m(t)$ determined by the correlator by the following equation:

$$C_m\left(t\right) = A + Be^{-2DK2m(t)}$$

where

A, B = constants dependent on the physical details of the measurement
K = the scattering constant for the eye which is $4\pi/\lambda(\sin\theta/2)$, where λ is the wavelength and θ is the scattering angle
t = the length of the predetermined time interval
m = an integer whose range is 1–64

Therefore, the values of the diffusion coefficient D and the constants A and B in the above equation can be determined, with the aid of computer 280, from the autocorrelation curve produced by the correlator 270 by using standard curve fitting and analysis techniques. The calculated diffusion coefficient can be stored in the computer along with other patient data including, in accordance with the invention, the patient's age.

The apparatus shown in Figs. 8.1 and 8.2 is used to perform a measurement of the lens diffusion coefficient as follows: with a patient sitting at the slit-lamp biomicroscope, the operator sets up the device in the same way that the device would be set up during a normal ophthalmic evaluation. In order to take measurements from various sites within the patient's lens, it is necessary that the pupil be dilated using routinely available dilating drops as normally used during the course of complete ophthalmic evaluation. Both the light produced by lamp 100 and the laser light with both filters in place are used to align the laser output as seen through the ocular 155 and 160 with the end of optical fiber light guide 195 in left ocular 155. Due to the standard adjustments on the biomicroscope and *XYZ* positioner 190, this alignment may be achieved at any desired site within the patient's lens.

Lamp 100 is then turned off and the operator depresses a foot switch which operates solenoid 203, sliding the movable filter in housing 215 out of the way to allow the actual measurement to be made using 1.5 mW laser light power. The second foot switch adjacent to the first can be used to turn laser 200 off should any emergency arise.

The back-scattered light output is measured by the photomultiplier through the optical system previously described and the photomultiplier output is processed as previously described by the photon correlation spectrometer. While measurements are in progress, the output of the spectrometer may be monitored by the oscilloscope connected to it. A measurement is made, for example, for 5 s at which point the first foot switch is released, reinserting the movable filter into the optical path, and concluding the measurement.

No contact lens, nor anesthetic drops are necessary to make a measurement. Although commonly used in eye examinations, anesthetic drops have various deleterious side effects. Such side effects include stinging, burning, and conjunctival redness as well as severe allergic reactions with resulting central nervous system stimulation or corneal damage. In addition, application of a contact lens following the use of a topical anesthetic requires much patient cooperation as well as experience on the part of the examiner. Further complications arising from the use of a contact lens include corneal abrasions and infection as well as recurrent and chronic corneal erosions. In contrast, the use of the apparatus disclosed herein is truly "noninvasive."

When employing the foregoing measurement technique to detect or monitor diabetes, a calculation of the diffusion coefficient s made on a series of patients whose health is known and are believed to be nondiabetic. The resulting measurements are compared to the patient's age resulting in a curve or graph similar to that shown in Fig. 8.3 (hypothetical measurements are shown for illustrative purposes). Figure 8.3 shows the value of the diffusion coefficient increasing in an upward direction along the vertical axis and patient age increasing rightward in the horizontal direction.

It has been discovered that patients who do not have diabetes (represented for example by points 300–305) all lie above a line (marked "normal" on the graph) while those patients suffering from diabetes lie below the line (represented by points 306–310). In addition, the severity of the disease is directly related to the distance below the line at which the measurement lies which increasing distance indicating increasing severity. For example, the patient represented by point 308 usually exhibits more severe symptoms than the patient represented by point 310.

After a curve such as that shown in Fig. 8.3 is obtained, patients can be screened for diabetes by making a measurement using the apparatus and method described above. The result of the measurement is then compared to Fig. 8.3. If the measurement is significantly below the "normal" line as shown in Fig. 8.3, the patient is likely to have diabetes or a disease which affects the lens similarly. Known diabetic patients can be monitored by making repeated measurements over a fixed period of time. The series of measurements are compared to the graph. An increasing distance from the "normal" line indicates an acceleration in the disease. A fixed distance indicates the disease that appears to be under reasonable control.

Although only one illustrative embodiment is shown of the invention, other changes and modifications within the spirit and scope of the invention will be apparent to those skilled in the art. Such modifications and changes are intended to be covered by the claims herein.

Chapter 9
Patents: Diabetes Detection Method #1

United States Patent	4,895,159
Weiss	**January 23, 1990**

Inventors:	**Weiss; Jeffrey N.** (Coconut Creek, FL)
Family ID:	27023442
Appl. No.:	06/672,717
Filed:	**November 19, 1984**

Related U.S. Patent Documents

Application Number	Filing Date	Patent Number	Issue Date
416654	Sep 10, 1982		

Current U.S. Class:	**600/558**; 600/316; 600/477
Current CPC Class:	A61B 3/1173 (20130101); A61B 5/14532 (20130101); A61B 5/1455 (20130101); A61B 5/411 (20130101); A61B 3/10 (20130101)
Current International Class:	A61B 3/117 (20060101); A61B 3/12 (20060101); A61B 5/00 (20060101); A61B 006/00 (); A61B 010/00 ()
Field of Search:	;128/633,745,664,665

© The Author(s), under exclusive license to Springer Nature
Switzerland AG 2022
J. N. Weiss, *Dynamic Light Scattering Spectroscopy of the Human Eye*,
https://doi.org/10.1007/978-3-031-06624-5_9

Other References

- Moses, "Alder's Physiology of the Eye", Sixth Ed., C. V. Mosby Co., St. Louis, 1975, pp. 275 and 287–295.
- *Primary Examiner*: Howell; Kyle L.
- *Assistant Examiner*: Hanley; John C.
- *Attorney, Agent or Firm*: Wolf, Greenfield & Sacks

Parent Case Text

Cross-reference to Related Applications

This application is a continuation-in-part of my parent patent application Ser. No. 416,654, filed Sept. 10, 1982, now abandoned. A divisional application of that parent application was filed on Nov. 15, 1984, and has been given Ser. No. 671,520.

Claims

I Claim

1. A method of screening a patient for diabetes mellitus comprises the following steps:

    A. Ascertaining the diffusion coefficient of the lens of the eye of each of a plurality of normal persons from variations in the intensity of light back-scattered from a clear site in the lens.
    B. Relating the ascertained diffusion coefficients with the respective ages of the normal persons to establish norms for nondiabetic persons of various ages.
    C. Ascertaining the diffusion coefficient of the lens of an in vivo eye of the patient from variations in the intensity of light back-scattered from a clear site in the lens.
    D. Determining whether the patient's diffusion coefficient is lower than the norm for nondiabetic persons of the same age as the patient.

2. The screening method according to claim I wherein step A comprises the following steps:

    (i)   Generating a light beam
    (ii) Focusing the light beam at a clear site in the nondiabetic person's lens
    (iii) Detecting variations in the light back-scattered from that site in the lens

3. The method according to claim 2 wherein step A further comprises the steps as follows:

(iv) Obtaining an autocorrelation function of the detected light variations
(v) Determining the diffusion coefficient from said autocorrelation function

4. The method according to claim 2 wherein step A further includes the step as follows:

(vi) Increasing the intensity of the light beam for the period in which variations in the light back-scattered from the lens are detected.

5. The screening method according to claim 1, wherein step C comprises the following steps:

(i) Generating a light beam
(ii) Focusing the light beam at a clear site in the lens of the patient's in vivo eye
(iii) Detecting variations in the light back-scattered from that clear site in the lens

6. The screening method according to claim 5, wherein step C further includes the step as follows:

(iv) Increasing the intensity of the light beam for the period in which variations in the light back-scattered from the lens are detected.

Description

Field of the Invention

This invention relates to medical diagnostic and monitoring methods and, in particular, to a method for detecting, diagnosing, and monitoring diabetes mellitus.

Background of the Invention

Diabetes mellitus is one of the leading causes of morbidity and mortality in the United States. Although the disease, once diagnosed, can be controlled, the diabetic patient faces many complications, some of them life-threatening. For example, the average life expectancy of the diabetic patient is one-third less than that of the general population; blindness is 25 times as common, renal disease is 17 times more common, gangrene is 5 times as common, and heart disease is twice as common in diabetics as compared to the nondiabetic.

In addition, the incidence of this disease appears to be increasing—between 1936 and 1978 there was a sixfold increase in the prevalence of the disease.

It is believed by many researchers in the field that many complications suffered by diabetic patients can be minimized or avoided by early detection of the onset of the disease and proper long-term control of the patient's blood glucose.

Unfortunately, prior art detection and monitoring methods have been unable to either accurately detect the onset of the disease at an early stage or assess the degree of control on a long-term basis. Such prior art detection methods, other than interpretation of clinical symptoms, rely on blood sugar measurements which reflect the presence of the disease. Prior art monitoring methods involve either spot blood sugar measurements or more complicated blood tests which reflect blood glucose levels that existed in the patient's body at a time 3 to 5 weeks prior to the time of measurement. Both prior art measurement methods require bodily invasion and the results are difficult to interpret.

Accordingly, it is an object of this invention to detect the onset of diabetes mellitus prior to the appearance of clinical symptoms.

It is another object of this invention to detect the development of diabetic eye disease.

It is still another object of this invention to assess the effectiveness of various methods of diabetic treatment.

It is yet another object of this invention to determine the relationship and degree of control required to prevent the occurrence of diabetic complications.

It is a further object of this invention to provide a method for objectively quantifying the effects of systemic disease, trauma, drugs, local inflammatory conditions of the eye, and aging.

Summary of the Invention

The foregoing objects are achieved from the ascertainment of the diffusion coefficient of the lens of a patient's in vivo eye by directing a beam of light from a low-power laser at a clear site in the lens of the patient's eye and measuring the intensity of the back-scattered light. A number of measurements are taken of the diffusion coefficient for patients known to be normal to establish a diffusion coefficient-age relationship. The ascertained lens diffusion coefficient of the patient is compared to the established relationship. Where a significant decrease of lens diffusion coefficient over the normal diffusion coefficient-age relationship is obtained, there is a likelihood that the patient is diabetic. The amount of decrease of lens diffusion coefficient over the normal established diffusion coefficient can be used as a measure of the severity of the disease or to monitor the progress and treatment of the disease.

The optical apparatus used in the performance of the method preferably consists of a low-power laser and associated optics attached to a slit-lamp biomicroscope equipped with precision mechanical adjustments to focus the light beam on the patient's lens. A photomultiplier is used to detect the intensity of the back-scattered light and a correlator is used to process the output of the photomultiplier to provide a set of numbers that can be used to calculate the diffusion coefficient.

Brief Description of the Drawings

Figure 8.1 is a perspective view of a slit-lamp biomicroscope and added equipment used to focus the light beam on the patient's lens

Figure 8.2 shows an overall schematic view of the optical arrangement to irradiate the patient's lens and the apparatus used to process the resulting signal

Figure 8.3 is a graph of lens diffusion coefficient versus patient age. The graph was developed from information obtained by using the apparatus described herein

Detailed Description of the Method

Figure 8.1 shows an optical arrangement for making measurements required in the performance of the method. That optical arrangement utilizes a modification of a commercially available instrument known as a slit-lamp biomicroscope. This device is well-known and is typically used in ophthalmological studies of the cornea, lens, and retina of the human eye. Slit-lamp biomicroscopes suitable for modification are manufactured by several companies and the operation and use of those devices are well-known to ophthalmologists and others engaged in the examination of human eyes.

Basically, a slit-lamp biomicroscope consists of a light source, a microscope, and a mechanical supporting arrangement that allows precise positioning of the light source and microscope relative to the patient to enable focusing of the light on selected portions of the patient's eye. Specifically, light produced by source 100 is reflected from mirror 105 and directed as beam 110 to the patient's eye shown schematically as eye 120. The apparatus also includes frame 115 and support 125 which position and hold the patient's head in a fixed position. Light which is reflected or scattered by the patient's cornea, lens, or retina, shown schematically as beam 130, is received by a binocular microscope arrangement 150 which has two eyepieces, 155 and 160. The lamp arrangement and microscope are supported by arms 140 and 145 from a common post, all in a well-known manner.

To facilitate making the requisite measurements, the standard slit-lamp biomicroscope is modified by the addition of an XYZ positioning apparatus to the microscope arrangement 150. In particular, the XYZ position apparatus consists of commercial XYZ positioner 190 which can obtain precise three-dimensional movement which is controlled by three orthogonal micrometers, 191–193. Positioner 190 is mounted on plate 194 which is in turn fastened to microscope arrangement 150 by means of a threaded hole 153 which is normally found on the arrangement and used for other purposes.

Attached to the movable surface of XYZ positioner 190 are arms 180 and 186 which support a lens arrangement 165. As will be hereinafter further explained, lens arrangement 165 is connected via fiber optic cable 170 to a laser and used to illuminate the patient's lens via beam 135. The back-scattered light shown schematically as beam 130 is detected by a sensor located in the focal plane of eyepiece 155 and conveyed via cable 195 to a photomultiplier (not shown).

Figure 8.2 of the drawings shows a schematic diagram of the preferred optical arrangement for making the measurements necessary to the performance of the method. The apparatus consists of a light source for illuminating a clear site in the lens of a patient's in vivo eye and a detecting or receiving portion for receiving the back-scattered radiation.

The light source part of the apparatus consists of laser 200, two filters mounted in housing 215, microscope objective lens 231, fiber optic termination 235, fiber optic cable 240, and focusing lens arrangement 245. Laser 200 is a 5-mW helium-neon laser of conventional design which is commercially available from several companies. A laser suitable for use with the illustrative embodiment is a model U-1305P, available from the Newport Corporation, 18235 Mount Baldy Circle, Fountain Valley, Calif. The output of laser 200 passes through two neutral density filters, mounted in housing 215. One filter is permanently mounted in the laser beam path and reduced the power output of laser 200 to 1.5 mW. The other filter is solenoid controlled so that it can automatically be moved out of the laser beam path during the measurement operation. When both filters are in place, they reduce the laser output power to 0.50 mW. The movable filter is used during premeasurement focusing, as will hereinafter be described, in order to reduce the patient's exposure to unnecessary laser irradiation. The movable filter is controlled by solenoid 203 which is under control of a footswitch operated by the person making the measurement. When solenoid 203 is operated, arm 220 retracts, in turn, sliding the movable filter in housing 215 by means of bell-crank 225.

After passing through one or both filters, the attenuated laser output light enters lens 231. Lens 231 is a 40× microscope objective lens which is mounted so that it focuses the laser light on the end of the optical fiber which transmits the light to the irradiating apparatus. Light passing through lens 231 falls onto an optical fiber 240 mounted in termination 235. The end of fiber 240 which enters termination 235 is attached to an *XYZ* positioner. The positioner is used to align the end of the optical fiber with the focusing lens to obtain maximum light transmission.

The other end of optical fiber 240 is attached to focusing lens arrangement 245. Lens arrangement 245 consists of a fiber optic holder which is slidably mounted in a lens holder tube. Lens 248 is a 18 mm focal-length converging lens which is mounted at the other end of the lens holder tube. The moveable arrangement between the fiber optic holder and the lens allows small adjustments to be made between the end of the optical fiber and the lens to permit fine focusing of the laser output beam at a given position within the patient's lens. Lens arrangement 245 is connected to the *XYZ* positioner attached to the slit-lamp biomicroscope as previously described and is used to focus the laser beam, 246, such that a sharp focus is achieved at a clear site in the patient's lens 250. After passing through the focal point in the lens, the beam becomes sharply defocused in order to maintain a low radiation level at the retina and prevent any possibility of injury or damage.

The detection optical system uses portions of the optical system of the slit-lamp biomicroscope. In particular, light back-scattered from the clear site in the patient's lens (represented schematically as beam 247) is focused by one objective of the binocular portion of microscope 255 onto a commercially available optical fiber light guide, 260, located at the center of the focal point of the eyepiece. In the illustrated embodiment, the end termination of optical fiber light guide 260 replaces the normal left ocular of slit-lamp biomicroscope 255. The arrangement is such that the end of fiber cable 260 can be seen when looking through the left ocular to allow focusing of the back-scattered radiation at the end of the fiber cable.

Scattered light received at microscope 255 is fed by fiber optic guide 260 to photomultiplier 210 which is a well-known, commercially available device. A photomultiplier suitable for use with the illustrative embodiment is a model number 9863B/350 manufactured by EMI Gencom, Inc., 80 Express Street, Plainview N.Y. The output of photomultiplier 210 is provided to amplifier-discriminator 265 which also is a well-known device that amplifies the output pulse signals produced by the photomultiplier and selectively sends to correlator 270 only those signals which have an amplitude above a preset threshold. A suitable amplifier-discriminator for use with the illustrated embodiment is a model number AD6 manufactured by Pacific Photometric Instruments, Inc., 5675 Landregan Street, Emeryville, Calif.

The output of amplifier-discriminator 265 is, in turn, provided to a commercial photon correlation spectrometer 270 (a suitable spectrometer is a model DC64 manufactured by Langley-Ford Instruments, 85 North Whitney Street, Amherst, Mass.). Correlator 270 counts the number of pulses received from amplifier-discriminator 265 for a predetermined time interval and performs a well-known mathematical operation to obtain the correlation function. A suitable time interval is 10 µs. The time interval, however, does not appear to be critical inasmuch as satisfactory measurements have been made in a time interval as short as 1.5 µs. The sample time may be chosen to further characterize the population of light scatterers. Measurements taken at shorter sample times, i.e., at 1.5 µs, appear to be more characteristic of smaller and/or faster scattering elements whereas measurements made at longer sample times, i.e., 200 µs, appear more characteristic of larger and/or slower scattering elements.

The correlator utilizes the received counts to solve the following equation for the autocorrelation function:

$$C_m(t) = \sum_{i=1}^{i=n} p_i p_i + m$$

where

t = the length of the predetermined time interval
i = an index number whose range is one to the total number of intervals
p_i = the number of pulses occurring during the ith time interval
n = the total number of intervals
m = an integer whose range is 1–64

In accordance with the above equation correlator 270 produces 64 solutions or points (one for each value of m) in a time sequence, each measurement separated by the value of t. These measurements may be plotted against time to produce a curve which may then be displayed for examination on oscilloscope 275. The values of the solutions may also be provided to computer 280 for further processing to determine the diffusion coefficient. A computer suitable for use with the illustrative embodiment is a personal computer manufactured by the International Business Machines Corporation, Armonk, N.Y.

In particular, the diffusion coefficient (D) is also related to the correlation function $C_m(t)$ determined by the correlator by the following equation:

$$C_m(t) = A + Be^{-2DK2m(t)}$$

where

A, B = constants dependent on the physical details of the measurement
K = the scattering constant for the eye which is $4\pi/\lambda(\sin\theta/2)$, where λ is the wavelength and θ is the scattering angle
t = the length of the predetermined time interval
m = an integer whose range is 1–64

Therefore, the values of the diffusion coefficient D and the constants A and B in the above equation can be determined, with the aid of computer 280, from the autocorrelation curve produced by the correlator 270 by using standard curve fitting and analysis techniques. The calculated diffusion coefficient can be stored in the computer along with other patient data including, in accordance with the invention, the patient's age.

The apparatus shown in Figs. 8.1 and 8.2 is used to perform a measurement of the lens diffusion coefficient as follows: with a patient sitting at the slit-lamp biomicroscope, the operator sets up the device in the same way that the device would be set up during a normal ophthalmic evaluation. In order to measure various positions within the periphery of the patient's lens, it is necessary that the pupil be dilated using routinely available dilating drops as normally used during the course of complete ophthalmic evaluation. Both the light produced by lamp 100 and the laser light with both filters in place are used to align the laser output as seen through the ocular 155 and 160 with the end of optical fiber light guide 195 in left ocular 155. Due to the standard adjustments on the biomicroscope and XYZ positioner 190, this alignment may be achieved at any selected site within the patient's lens. The operator selects a site that is clear, i.e., a site that is free of opacities.

Lamp 100 is then turned off and the operator depresses a foot switch which operates solenoid 203 sliding the movable filter in housing 215 out of the way to allow the actual measurement to be made using 1.5 mW laser light power. The second foot switch adjacent to the first can be used to turn laser 200 off should any emergency arise.

The back-scattered light output is measured by the photomultiplier through the optical system previously described and the photomultiplier output is processed as previously described by the photon correlation spectrometer. While measurements are in progress, the output of the spectrometer may be monitored by the oscilloscope connected to it. A measurement is made, for example, for 5 s at which point the first foot switch is released, reinserting the movable filter into the optical path, and concluding the measurement.

When performing the method to screen for diabetes mellitus, measurements are taken only from "clear" sites in the lens of the eye. That is, measurements are taken only from sites in the lens that are non-opaque. The yellowing of the lens that is normal in the human aging process is deemed not to be an opacity. In normal humans, discernable yellowing of the lens first appears at about 30 years of age and thereafter that yellowing tends to increase with age. Measurements taken from cataracts (i.e., from opacities in the lens) are deemed, at this time, to be unreliable because sufficient information has not yet been developed from clinical studies to enable such measurements to be linked with any certainty to diabetes mellitus.

In order to accurately compare measurements made from an individual with measurements made from the same individual at a later time or with measurements from a different individual, the compared measurements should be made from approximately the same position in the lens. Measurements obtained from other positions in the lens may give somewhat different results which can provide additional information concerning the health of the patient. For standardization purposes, it has been my practice to take measurements from a non-opaque site in the central nucleus of the lens.

By using the apparatus described herein, no contact lens, nor anesthetic drops are necessary to make a measurement. Although commonly used in eye examinations, anesthetic drops have various deleterious side effects. Such side effects include stinging, burning, and conjunctival redness as well as severe allergic reactions with resulting central nervous system stimulation or corneal damage. In addition, application of a contact lens following the use of a topical anesthetic requires much patient cooperation as well as experience on the part of the examiner. Further complications arising from the use of a contact lens include corneal abrasions and infection as well as recurrent and chronic corneal erosions. In contrast, by employing the described apparatus, the method can truly be "noninvasive."

In using the method to detect and monitor diabetes, a calculation of the diffusion coefficient is made on a series of patients whose health is known and are believed to be nondiabetic. The resulting measurements are compared to the patient's age resulting in a curve or graph similar to that shown in Fig. 8.3 (hypothetical measurements are shown for illustrative purposes). Figure 8.3 shows the value of the diffusion coefficient increasing in an upward direction along the vertical axis and patient age increasing rightward in the horizontal direction.

It has been discovered that the diffusion coefficient for patients who do not have diabetes (represented for example by points 300–305) all lie above a line (marked "normal" on the graph) while the diffusion coefficient for patients having diabetes lie below the line (represented by points 306–310). In addition, the severity of the

disease is directly related to the distance below the line at which the ascertained diffusion coefficient lies, with increasing distance indicating greater severity. For
example, the patient represented by point 308 usually exhibits more severe symptoms than the patient represented by point 310.

When a curve such as that shown in Fig. 8.3 has been established, patients can be
screened for diabetes by comparing their ascertained diffusion coefficients with the
"normal" line. If the measurement is significantly below the "normal" line as shown
in Fig. 8.3, the patient is likely to have diabetes or a disease which affects the lens
similarly. Known diabetic patients can be monitored by making repeated measurements over a fixed period of time. The series of measurements are compared to the
graph. An increasing distance from the "normal" line indicates an acceleration in
the disease. A fixed distance indicates the disease that appears to be under reasonable control.

Changes and modifications within the spirit and scope of the invention will be
apparent to those skilled in the art. I have, for example, found that measurements of
back-scattered light may also be taken from the cornea or the retina of the eye.
However, measurements taken from the lens have thus far given the best results. As
another example the diffusion coefficient can be replaced by an equivalent measure
such as the decay constant. The essential point is that variations in the intensity of
the back scattered light is utilized to obtain a measurement. That measurement may
then be used to obtain derivatives. Such modifications and changes are intended to
be covered by the claims herein.

Chapter 10
Patents: Diabetes Detection Method #2

United States Patent	5,025,785
Weiss	June 25, 1991

Inventors:	Weiss; Jeffrey N. (Coconut Creek, FL)
Family ID:	27411105
Appl. No.:	07/418,109
Filed:	October 6, 1989

Related U.S. Patent Documents

Application Number	Filing Date	Patent Number	Issue Date
672717	Nov 19, 1984	4895159	Jan 23, 1990
416654	Sep 10, 1982		

Current U.S. Class:	600/318; 128/898; 600/477
Current CPC Class:	A61B 3/1173 (20130101); A61B 3/1225 (20130101); A61B 5/14532 (20130101); A61B 5/411 (20130101)
Current International Class:	A61B 3/117 (20060101); A61B 3/12 (20060101); A61B 5/00 (20060101); A61B 006/00 ()
Field of Search:	;128/633,634,665,898

© The Author(s), under exclusive license to Springer Nature
Switzerland AG 2022
J. N. Weiss, *Dynamic Light Scattering Spectroscopy of the Human Eye*,
https://doi.org/10.1007/978-3-031-06624-5_10

References Cited [Referenced by]

U.S. Patent Documents

4715703	December 1987	Cornsweet et al.

- *Primary Examiner*: Hindenburg; Max
- *Assistant Examiner*: Shay; David
- *Attorney, Agent or Firm*: Wolf, Greenfield & Sacks

Parent Case Text

Cross-reference to Related Applications

This application is a continuation-in-part of my application Ser. No. 672,717, now U.S. Pat. No. 4,895,159, issued Jan. 23, 1990. That earlier application is a continuation-in-art of my parent patent application Ser. No. 416,654, which was filed on Sept. 10, 1982, and is now abandoned. Before that parent application was abandoned, a divisional patent application Ser. No. 671,520 was filed on Nov. 15, 1984, and became U.S. Pat. No. 4,883,351 issued on Nov. 28, 1989. Applicant incorporates by reference into this application all of the specifications and claims of said earlier application and U.S. Pat. Nos. 4,895,159, 416,654, and 4,883,351.

Claims

What is claimed is:

1. A noninvasive method of examining a patient for diabetes mellitus, comprising the following steps:

   A. Ascertaining the variations in the intensity of light back-scattered from the cornea of an in vivo eye of each of a plurality of normal persons and deriving measurements therefrom.
   B. Relating the derived measurements with the respective ages of the normal persons to obtain norms for persons of various ages.
   C. Ascertaining the variations in the intensity of the light back-scattered from the cornea a corresponding measurement therefrom.
   D. Comparing the patient's measurement with the norm for persons of comparable age to the patient.

2. The method according to claim 1, wherein the measurements are made from the same layer of the cornea of the in vivo eyes of the patient and the normal persons.
3. A noninvasive method of examining a patient for diabetes mellitus, comprising the steps as follows:

A. Ascertaining the variations in the intensity of light back-scattered from the conjunctiva of the in vivo eye of each of a plurality of normal persons and deriving measurements therefrom.
B. Relating the derived measurements with the respective ages of the normal persons to obtain norms for persons of various ages.
C. Ascertaining the variations in the intensity of light back-scattered from the conjunctiva of the patient's in vivo eye and deriving corresponding measurements therefrom.
D. Comparing the patient's measurements with the norm for persons of comparable age to the patient.

4. A noninvasive method of examining a patient for diabetes mellitus, comprising the steps as follows:

A. Ascertaining the variations in the intensity of light back-scattered from the retina of the in vivo eye of each of a plurality of normal persons and deriving measurements therefrom.
B. Relating the derived measurements with the respective ages of the normal persons to obtain norms for persons of various ages.
C. Ascertaining the variations in the intensity of light back-scattered from the retina of the patient's in vivo eye and deriving corresponding measurements therefrom.
D. Comparing the patient's measurements with the norm for persons of comparable age to the patient.

Description

Field of the Invention

This invention relates to medical diagnostic and monitoring methods and, in particular, to a method for detecting, diagnosing, and monitoring diabetes mellitus.

Background of the Invention

Diabetes mellitus is one of the leading causes of morbidity and mortality in the United States. Although the disease, once diagnosed, can be controlled, the diabetic patient faces many complications, some of them life threatening. For example, the average life expectancy of the diabetic patient is one-third less than that of the general population; blindness is 25 times as common, renal disease is 17 times more common, gangrene is 5 times as common, and heart disease is twice as common in diabetics as compared to the nondiabetic.

In addition, the incidence of this disease appears to be increasing—between 1936 and 1978 there was a sixfold increase in the prevalence of the disease.

It is believed by many researchers in the field that many complications suffered by diabetic patients can be minimized or avoided by early detection of the onset of the disease and proper long-term control of the patient's blood glucose.

Unfortunately, prior art detection and monitoring methods have been unable to either accurately detect the onset of the disease at an early stage or assess the degree of control on a long-term basis. Such prior art detection methods, other than interpretation of clinical symptoms, rely on blood sugar measurements which reflect the presence of the disease. Prior art monitoring methods involve either spot blood sugar measurements or more complicated blood tests which reflect blood glucose levels that existed in the patient's body at a time 3–5 weeks prior to the time of measurement. Both prior art measurement methods require bodily invasion and the results are difficult to interpret.

Accordingly, it is an objective of this invention to detect the onset of diabetes mellitus prior to the appearance of clinical symptoms.

It is another object of this invention to detect the development of diabetic eye disease.

It is still another object of this invention to assess the effectiveness of various methods of diabetic treatment.

It is yet another object of this invention to determine the relationship and degree of control required to prevent the occurrence of diabetic complications.

It is a further object of this invention to provide a method for objectively quantifying the effects of systemic disease, trauma, drugs, local inflammatory conditions of the eye, and aging.

Summary of the Invention

The foregoing objects are achieved from the ascertainment of the diffusion coefficient of the lens of a patient's in vivo eye by directing a beam of light from a low-power laser at a clear site in the lens of the patient's eye and measuring the intensity of the hack-scattered light. A number of measurements are taken of the diffusion coefficient for patients known to be normal to establish a diffusion coefficient-age relationship. The ascertained lens diffusion coefficient of the patient is compared to the established relationship. Where a significant decrease of lens diffusion coefficient over the normal diffusion coefficient-age relationship is obtained, there is a likelihood that the patient is diabetic. The amount of decrease of lens diffusion coefficient over the normal established diffusion coefficient can be used as a measure of the severity of the disease or to monitor the progress and treatment of the disease.

In lieu of or in addition to making measurements from the lens of the patient's in vivo eye, measurements may be taken from the conjunctiva, the cornea, and the retina of the patient's eye. Those parts of the eye are appreciably affected by diabetes mellitus in addition to the lens of the eye. Because measurements taken from the lens have thus far provided the best results, the invention is here described with the taking of measurements only from the lens of the eye. From that description, the extension of the measurement technique to the conjunctiva, cornea, or retina is self-evident.

The optical apparatus used in the performance of the method preferably consists of a low-power laser and associated optics attached to a slit-lamp biomicroscope equipped with precision mechanical adjustments to focus the light beam on the patient's lens. A photomultiplier is used to detect the intensity of the back-scattered light and a correlator is used to process the output of the photomultiplier to provide a set of numbers that can be used to calculate the diffusion coefficient.

Brief Description of the Drawings

Figure 8.1 is a perspective view of a slit-lamp biomicroscope and added equipment used to focus the light beam on the patient's lens

Figure 8.2 shows an overall schematic view of the optical arrangement to irradiate the patient's lens and the apparatus used to process the resulting signal

Figure 8.3 is a graph of lens diffusion coefficient versus patient age. The graph was developed from information obtained by using the apparatus described herein

Detailed Description of the Method

Figure 8.1 shows an optical arrangement for making measurements required in the performance of the method. That optical arrangement utilizes a modification of a commercially available instrument known as a slit-lamp biomicroscope. This device is well known and is typically used in ophthalmological studies of the conjunctiva, cornea, lens, and retina of the human eye. Slit-lamp biomicroscopes suitable for modification are manufactured by several companies and the operation and use of those devices are well-known to ophthalmologists and others engaged in the examination of human eyes.

Basically, a slit-lamp biomicroscope consists of a light source, a microscope, and a mechanical supporting arrangement that allows precise positioning of the light source and microscope relative to the patient to enable focusing of the light on selected portions of the patient's eye. Specifically, light produced by source 100 is reflected from mirror 105 and directed as beam 110 to the patient's eye shown schematically an eye 120. The apparatus also includes frame 115 and support 125 which position and hold the patient's head in a fixed position. Light which is reflected or scattered by the patient's conjunctiva, cornea, lens, or retina, shown schematically as beam 130, is received by a binocular microscope arrangement 150 which has two eyepieces, 155 and 160. The lamp arrangement and microscope are supported by arms 140 and 145 from a common post, all in a well-known manner.

To facilitate making the requisite measurements, the standard slit-lamp biomicroscope is modified by the addition of an *XYZ* positioning apparatus to the microscope arrangement 150. In particular, the *XYZ* position apparatus consists of commercial *XYZ* positioner 190 which can obtain precise three-dimensional movement which is controlled by three orthogonal micrometers, 191–193. Positioner 190 is mounted on plate 194 which is in turn fastened to microscope arrangement 150 by means of a threaded hole 153 which is normally found on the arrangement and used for other purposes.

Attached to the movable surface of *XYZ* positioner 190 are arms 180 and 186 which support a lens arrangement 165. As will be hereinafter further explained, lens arrangement 165 is connected via fiber optic cable 170 to a laser and used to illuminate the patient's lens via beam 135. The back-scattered light shown schematically as beam 130 is detected by a sensor located in the focal plane of eyepiece 155 and conveyed via cable 195 to a photomultiplier (not shown).

Figure 8.2 of the drawings shows a schematic diagram of the preferred optical arrangement for making the measurements necessary to the performance of the method. The apparatus consists of a light source for illuminating a clear site in the lens of a patient's in vivo eye and a detecting or receiving portion for receiving the back scattered radiation.

The light source part of the apparatus consists of laser 200, two filters mounted in housing 215, microscope objective lens 231, fiber optic termination 235, fiber optic cable 240, and focusing lens arrangement 245. Laser 200 is a 5-mW helium-neon laser of conventional design which is commercially available from several companies. A laser suitable for use with the illustrative embodiment is a model U-1305P, available from the Newport Corporation, 18235 Mount Baldy Circle, Fountain Valley, Calif. The output of laser 200 passes through two neutral density filters, mounted in housing 215. One filter is permanently mounted in the laser beam path and reduced the power output of laser 200 to 1.5 mW. The other filter is solenoid-controlled so that it can automatically be moved out of the laser beam path during the measurement operation. When both filters are in place, they reduce the laser output power to 0.50 mW. The movable filter is used during premeasurement focusing, as will hereinafter be described, in order to reduce the patient's exposure to unnecessary laser irradiation. The movable filter is controlled by solenoid 203 which is under control of a footswitch operated by the person making the measurement. When solenoid 203 is operated, arm 220 retracts, in turn, sliding the movable filter in housing 215 by means of bell crank 225.

After passing through one or both filters, the attenuated laser output light enters lens 231. Lens 231 is a 40× microscope objective lens which is mounted so that it focuses the laser light on the end of the optical fiber which transmits the light to the irradiating apparatus. Light passing through lens 231 falls onto an optical fiber 240 mounted in termination 235. The end of fiber 240 which enters termination 235 is attached to an *XYZ* positioner. The positioner is used to align the end of the optical fiber with the focusing lens to obtain maximum light transmission.

The other end of optical fiber 240 is attached to focusing lens arrangement 245. Lens arrangement 245 consists of a fiber optic holder which is slidably mounted in a lens holder tube. Lens 248 is an 18 mm focal-length converging lens which is mounted at the other end of the lens holder tube. The movable arrangement between the fiber optic holder and the lens allows small adjustments to be made between the end of the optical fiber and the lens to permit fine focusing of the laser output beam at a given position within the patient's lens. Lens arrangement 245 is connected to the *XYZ* positioner attached to the slit-lamp biomicroscope as previously described and is used to focus the laser beam, 246, such that a sharp focus is achieved at a clear site in the patient's lens 250. After passing through the focal point in the lens the beam becomes sharply defocused in order to maintain a low radiation level at the retina and prevent any possibility of injury or damage.

The detection optical system uses portions of the optical system of the slit-lamp biomicroscope. In particular, light back-scattered from the clear site in the patient s lens (represented schematically as beam 247) is focused by one objective of the binocular portion of microscope 255 onto a commercially available optical fiber light guide, 260, located at the center of the focal point of the eyepiece. In the illus-trated embodiment, the end termination of optical fiber light guide 260 replaces the normal left ocular of slit-lamp biomicroscope 255. The arrangement is such that the end of fiber cable 260 can be seen when looking through the left ocular to allow focusing of the back-scattered radiation on the end of the fiber cable.

Scattered light received at microscope 255 is fed by fiber optic guide 260 to pho-tomultiplier 210 which is a well-known, commercially available device. A photo-multiplier suitable for use with the illustrative embodiment is a model number 9863B/350 manufactured by EMI Gencom, Inc., 80 Express Street, Plainview, N.Y. The output of photomultiplier 210 is provided to amplifier-discriminator 265 which also is a well-known device that amplifies the output pulse signals produced by the photomultiplier and selectively sends to correlator 270 only those signals which have an amplitude above a preset threshold. A suitable amplifier-discriminator for use with the illustrated embodiment is a model number AD6 manufactured by Pacific Photometric Instruments Inc., 5675 Landregan Street. Emeryville, Calif.

The output of amplifier-discriminator 265 is, in turn, provided to a commercial photon correlation spectrometer 270 (a suitable spectrometer is a model DC64 man-ufactured by Langley-Ford Instruments, 85 North Whitney Street, Amherst, Mass.). Correlator 270 counts the number of pulses received from amplifier-discriminator 265 for a predetermined time interval and performs a well-known mathematical operation to obtain the correlation function. A suitable time interval is 10 μs. The sample time may be chosen to further characterize the population of light scatterers. Measurements taken at shorter sample times, i.e., at 1.5 μs, appear to be more char-acteristic of smaller and/or faster scattering elements whereas measurements made at longer sample times, i.e., 200 μs, appear more characteristic of larger and/or slower scattering elements.

The correlator utilizes the received counts to solve the following equation for the autocorrelation function:

$$C_m(t) = \sum_{i=1}^{i=n} p_i p_i + m$$

where

t = the length of the predetermined time interval
i = an index number whose range is one to the total number of intervals
p_i = the number of pulses occurring during the ith time interval
n = the total number of intervals
m = an integer whose range is 1–64

In accordance with the above equation, correlator 270 produces 64 solutions or points (one for each value of m) in a time sequence, each measurement separated by the value of t. These measurements may be plotted against time to produce a curve which may then be displayed for examination on oscilloscope 275. The values of the solutions may also be provided to computer 280 for further processing to determine the diffusion coefficient. A computer suitable for use with the illustrative embodiment is a personal computer manufactured by the International Business Machines Corporation. Armonk, New York.

In particular, the diffusion coefficient (D) is also related to the correlation function $C_m(t)$ determined by the correlator by the following equation:

$$C_m(t) = A + Be^{-2DK2m(t)}$$

where

A, B = constants dependent on the physical details of the measurement
K = the scattering constant for the eye which is $4\pi/\lambda(\sin\theta/2)$ where λ is the wavelength and θ is the scattering angle
t = the length of the predetermined time interval
m = an integer whose range is 1–64

Therefore, the values of the diffusion coefficient D and the constants A and B in the above equation can be determined, with the aid of computer 280, from the autocorrelation curve produced by the correlator 270 by using standard curve fitting and analysis techniques. The calculated diffusion coefficient can be stored in the computer along with other patient data, including, in accordance with the invention, the patient's age.

The apparatus shown in Figs. 8.1 and 8.2 is used to perform a measurement of the lens diffusion coefficient as follows: with a patient sitting at the slit-lamp biomicroscope, the operator sets up the device in the same way that the device would be set up during a normal ophthalmic evaluation. In order to measure various positions within the periphery of the patient's lens, it is necessary that the pupil be dilated using routinely available dilating drops as normally used during the course of complete ophthalmic evaluation. Both the light produced by lamp 100 and the laser light with both filters in place are used to align the laser output as seen through the ocular 155 and 160 with the end of optical fiber light guide 195 in left ocular 155. Due to the standard adjustments on the biomicroscope and *XYZ* positioner 190, this alignment may be achieved at any selected site within the patient's lens. The operator selects a site that is clear, i.e., a site that is free of opacities.

Lamp 100 is then turned off and the operator depresses a foot switch which operates solenoid 203 sliding the movable filter in housing 215 out of the way to allow the actual measurement to be made using 1.5 mW laser light power. The second foot switch adjacent to the first can be used to turn laser 200 off should any emergency arise.

The back-scattered light output is measured by the photomultiplier through the optical system previously described and the photomultiplier output is processed as previously described by the photon correlation spectrometer. While measurements are in progress, the output of the spectrometer may be monitored by the oscilloscope connected to it. A measurement is made, for example, for 5 s at which point the first foot switch is released, reinserting the movable filter into the optical path, and concluding the measurement.

When performing the method to screen for diabetes mellitus, measurements are taken only from "clear" sites in the lens of the eye. That is, measurements are taken only from sites in the lens that are non-opaque. The yellowing of the lens that is normal in the human aging process is deemed not to be an opacity. In normal humans, discernable yellowing of the lens first appears at about 30 years of age and thereafter that yellowing tends to increase with age. Measurements taken from cataracts (i.e., from opacities in the lens) are deemed, at this time, to be unreliable because sufficient information has not yet been developed from clinical studies to enable such measurements to be linked with any certainty to diabetes mellitus.

In order to accurately compare measurements made from an individual with measurements made from the same individual at a later time or with measurements from a different individual, the compared measurements should be made from approximately the same position in the lens. Measurements obtained from other positions in the lens may give somewhat different results which can provide additional information concerning the health of the patient. For standardization purposes, it has been my practice to take measurements from a non-opaque site in the central nucleus of the lens.

By using the apparatus described herein, no contact lens, nor anesthetic drops are necessary to make a measurement. Although commonly used in eye examinations, anesthetic drops have various deleterious side effects. Such side effects include stinging, burning, and conjunctival redness as well as severe allergic reactions with resulting central nervous system stimulation or corneal damage. In addition, application of a contact lens following the use of a topical anesthetic requires much patient cooperation as well as experience on the part of the examiner. Further complications arising from the use of a contact lens include corneal abrasions and infection as well as recurrent and chronic corneal erosions. In contrast, by employing the described apparatus, the method can truly be "noninvasive."

In using the method to detect and monitor diabetes, a calculation of the diffusion coefficient is made on a series of patients whose health is known and are believed to be nondiabetic. The resulting measurements are compared to the patient's age resulting in a curve or graph similar to that shown in Fig. 8.3 (hypothetical measurements are shown for illustrative purposes). Figure 8.3 shows the value of the diffusion coefficient increasing in an upward direction along the vertical axis and patient age increasing rightward in the horizontal direction.

It has been discovered that the diffusion coefficient for patients who do not have diabetes (represented for example by points 300–305) all lie above a line (marked "normal" on the graph) while the diffusion coefficient for patients having diabetes lie below the line (represented by points 306–310). In addition, the severity of the disease is directly related to the distance below the line at which the ascertained diffusion coefficient lies, with increasing distance indicating greater severity. For example, the patient represented by point 308 usually exhibits more severe symptoms than the patient represented by point 310.

When a curve such as that shown in Fig. 8.3 has been established, patients can be screened for diabetes by comparing their ascertained diffusion coefficients with the "normal" line If the measurement is significantly below the "normal" line as shown in Fig. 8.3 the patient is likely to have diabetes or a disease which affects the lens similarly. Known diabetic patients can be monitored by making repeated measurements over a fixed period of time. The series of measurements are compared to the graph. An increasing distance from the "normal" line indicates an acceleration in the disease. A fixed distance indicates the disease appears to be under reasonable control.

I have found that measurements of back-scattered light may be taken from the conjunctiva, the cornea, and the retina of the eye. Those parts of the eye are appreciably affected by the presence of diabetes mellitus in addition to the lens of the eye. Thus far, however, measurements taken from the lens have given the best results. When measurements are taken from the cornea, it is important for comparison purposes, to take the measurements from the same layer of the cornea. The layers of the cornea (the epithelium, for example) are thin and care must be exercised to assure that the measurements are taken from the desired layer. Consequently, depth perception, when setting up and taking the measurements, is a requirement that must be strictly observed. For comparison purposes, it is preferred to take the measurements from approximately the same site in the layer. In this respect, however, that requirement is not as critical as when measurements are made from the lens. That is, considerable variation in the sites from which measurements are taken is permissible when measurements are taken from the cornea.

Where measurements are taken from the conjunctiva or from the retina, it is preferable to take the measurements from the surface at the front of conjunctiva or retina. Depth perception is important to assure that the measurements are taken from the front surface of the retina or conjunctiva. To prevent damage to the retina, low intensity light should be used. As with the cornea, it is not as critical, for comparison purposes, to take the measurements from the same site on the retina, cornea, or the conjunctiva as it is when measurements are taken from the lens.

Changes and modifications within the spirit and scope of the invention will be apparent to those skilled in ophthalmology. As an example, the diffusion coefficient can be replaced by an equivalent measure such as the decay constant. The essential point is that variations in the intensity of the back-scattered light are the basis of the measurement. That measurement may then be utilized to obtain derivatives. The form in which those variations are presented is mainly a matter of individual preference. Such obvious modifications and changes are intended to be covered by the appended claims.

Chapter 11
Patents: Filed Patent Application— Apparatus and Method for the Detection of Dementia and Retinal Conditions

This application claims priority to and the benefit of U.S. Application Serial No. 62/622,775, filed January 26, 2018, which application is incorporated by reference in its entirety for all purposes.

This application also incorporates by reference U.S. Application Serial No. 61/475,030, filed April 13, 2011 in its entirety.

Field of the Invention

This invention relates to medical diagnostic and monitoring methods and, in particular, to a method for the detection and monitoring of dementia and the effectiveness of potential therapies.

Background of the Invention

Dementia is a common cause of morbidity and mortality. It is caused by physical changes in the brain that causes the loss of mental abilities and memory that affect the activities of daily living. The types of dementia include: Alzheimer's disease, Vascular dementia, Dementia with Lewy bodies, Mixed dementia, Parkinson's disease, Frontotemporal dementia, Creutzfeld-Jakob disease, Normal pressure hydrocephalus, Huntington's disease, Wernicke-Korsakoff Syndrome, etc.

Alzheimer's disease is a slowly progressive brain disease beginning prior to the appearance of symptoms and accounts for approximately 60–80% of dementia cases. Definitive diagnosis is made posthumously with the discovery of protein fragment beta-amyloid plaques and twisted strands of the protein tau (tangles) with nerve cell damage and death.

© The Author(s), under exclusive license to Springer Nature
Switzerland AG 2022
J. N. Weiss, *Dynamic Light Scattering Spectroscopy of the Human Eye*,
https://doi.org/10.1007/978-3-031-06624-5_11

Vascular dementia, previously known as post-stroke or multi-infarct dementia is solely diagnosed in approximately 10% of dementia cases. The development of Lewy bodies in the cerebral cortex can cause dementia. The type of aggregate pattern may be indicative of Dementia with Lewy bodies or of Parkinson's disease.

Abnormalities of more than one dementia cause may occur simultaneously in the brain causing a mixed dementia. In Parkinson's disease the alpha-synuclein clumps generally occur in a deep area of the brain called the substantia nigra and are thought to affect the production of dopamine.

In Normal Pressure Hydrocephalus, an abnormal increase of fluid in the brain leads to dementia. This may sometimes be corrected by the placement of a shunt in the brain to drain the excess fluid. There are no definite distinguishing microscopic abnormalities seen in all cases of frontotemporal dementia.

Creutzfeldt-Jakob disease (mad-cow disease) is caused by an infection with a prion. Huntington's disease is caused by a defective gene on chromosome 4. Vitamin B-1 deficiency (thiamine), generally caused by alcoholism, is the cause of Wernicke-Korsakoff syndrome.

In the absence of dementia etiology, as seen in Creutzfeldt-Jakob disease, Normal Pressure Hydrocephalus, Huntington's disease, Wernicke-Korsakoff syndrome, the true diagnosis is generally made pathologically, after the patient has expired.

During the last 15 years, there have been more than 400 clinical trials of therapeutic agents for Alzheimer's disease registered with the National Institute of Health website, clinicaltrials.gov. For those trials with reported results, the failure rate has been almost 100%. Though most trials typically last 1.5–3 years, it has been estimated that, depending on the efficacy of the therapeutic intervention, study duration would need to be 5–10 years in duration to detect an effect.

Therefore, what is needed is a sensitive, quantitative, technique that can detect the beginnings or early onset of these conditions before the development of symptoms.

The retina is visible within the eye and is composed of nine histologic layers. The nerve fiber layer of the retina is an extension of the brain. The early detection of neurologic damage at the microscopic level when it is still potentially reversible is a prerequisite for the development of potential cures. The early detection of the effectiveness of treatment allows for better and more effective treatments.

It has been demonstrated that patients with Alzheimer's disease have thinning of the retinal nerve fiber layer and retinal ganglion cell layer by ocular coherence tomography (OCT) images and measurements taken through the macula and peripapillary areas. This was consistent with histopathologic data. Inner retina thinning has been correlated with disease severity. This may be related to the presence of amyloid-beta within the retina.

Inner retinal thinning has been found in other neurodegenerative diseases including multiple sclerosis, amyotrophic lateral sclerosis, dementia with Lewy bodies, and multiple system atrophy.

As compared to the inner retinal thinning seen in Alzheimer's disease, thinning of the photoreceptor or outer retina thinning has been found in frontotemporal degeneration. Approximately 30% of patients initially diagnosed with frontotemporal degeneration are subsequently diagnosed with Alzheimer's disease at autopsy.

Dynamic Light Scattering, also known as Photon Correlation Spectroscopy (PCS), a technique which measures the scattered light intensity fluctuations resulting from the thermal random motion (Brownian motion), has been used to predict the development of cataractogenesis in rabbits, and detect the development of cataract formation and of diabetes mellitus in humans. The results demonstrated the utility of PCS to noninvasively quantitate subtle changes at the molecular level.

The present invention is directed to addressing the need for a sensitive, quantitative technique that can detect the beginnings or early onset of these conditions before the development of symptoms.

Summary of the Invention

Accordingly, it is an object of this invention to detect the onset of neurologic disease before the onset of clinical symptoms.

It is another object of this invention to study the effectiveness of various medications on the neurologic disease.

It is a further object of this invention to provide a method where the appropriate threshold or time for the delivery of the therapeutic intervention to be the most efficacious may be discovered.

Another object of this invention is to monitor the effectiveness of therapeutic interventions to treat ophthalmic conditions and diseases.

The foregoing objects are achieved from the calculation of the diffusion coefficient from the retina of a patient's in vivo eye by directing a beam of light from a low-power laser or other coherent light source at a spot in the retina or choroid of the patient's eye and measuring the fluctuations in the intensity of the back-scattered light. A number of measurements are taken from the retina or choroid of normal or disease-free patients of similar ages to establish a database, such as but not limited to, an electronic database, for comparison with the abnormal results. In addition, or alternatively, the subject may be analyzed over time to determine changes in the measurement from an initial or baseline measurement or taken before and after a therapeutic intervention. The diffusion coefficient or another calculated term may be used to diagnose, measure the severity of the disease, monitor the progress and treatment of the condition, or assess the efficacy of therapeutic interventions. The measurement may be utilized with or compared with an Ocular Coherence Tomography (OCT) image and measurement also made from the same or nearby area of the retina.

The apparatus used to perform this method may include a low-power laser or other coherent light source and associated optics attached to a commercially available fundus camera. Utilizing the optical pathway of the fundus camera precludes the necessity of using a contact lens to focus light on the retina. A flat contact lens may be used to stabilize the eye and prevent eye movement during the measurement but is not considered necessary.

An infrared viewing light may be used to aid in the maintenance of the measuring spot on a specific area of the retina or choroid when the visible light of the fundus camera is deactivated during the performance of the measurement. An automatic focusing and alignment system may be utilized. The location chosen for measurement may also be made on the basis of fundus autofluorescence, fundus fluorescein angiography, OCT, or another imaging technology.

The device may be incorporated with or within an OCT device so at one sitting, both measurements/tests may be made from the patient. A digital photon counter is used to detect fluctuations in the intensities of the back-scattered light and a digital correlator is used to process the output of the photon counter to provide a set of numbers that can be used to calculate the diffusion coefficient or another mathematical term.

As part of the diagnostic process, patients undergo an ophthalmic examination to exclude confounding eye diseases. An OCT image and measurement is taken to aid in the determination and location of retinal thickness and to exclude pathology that would affect the DLS measurement. A cognition test, such as a Mini-Mental State Exam may also be performed.

Brief Description of the Drawings

Figure 8.1 shows a non-limiting embodiment of the electronic components in accordance with the present disclosure

Figure 8.2 illustrates a non-limiting attachment of the optical system to the fundus camera

Figure 8.3 details a non-limiting embodiment of the electrical components in accordance with the present disclosure

Detailed Description

In Fig. 8.1, the light source part of the apparatus can consist of laser 200, laser safety threshold circuit 205, and shutter assemblies 210 and 215. Laser 200 can be an approximately 1.5-mW helium-neon laser of conventional design that is commercially available from several companies. The laser output provides an optical power to the patient below the maximal permissible exposure recommended by the American National Standards Institute, ANSI Z136.1 (2014) standard. The minimal amount of light necessary to make a successful measurement is used and may be determined by experimentation.

In Fig. 8.2, light passing through optical fiber 220 is mounted in termination 225 that is attached to a linear positioner 230 on the fundus camera attachment 235. The positioner is available to vary the measurement spot on the retina. Mirrors 240, 245, and a beam splitter 250 are provided to place the incident beam into the frame of the fundus camera image of the retina.

The detection optical fiber 255 attached to the linear positioner 230 on the fundus camera so both the incident light and detection light is simultaneously varied by the same amount. The light output of detection fiber 255 is detected by single photon counting module 260 and processed by the correlator software on a personal computer.

Optics may be incorporated to vary the diameter of the beam on the retina or choroid thus allowing a greater or smaller area to be sampled or measured. Modifications may also be made to the detection fiberoptic such that a smaller or larger measurement area may be made.

The optical arrangement is attached to a frame that is easily attached to a commercially available instrument known as a fundus camera. This device is well-known and is typically used in ophthalmological studies of the eye. Fundus cameras suitable for modification are manufactured by several companies and the conventional operation and use of those devices are well-known to ophthalmologists and others engaged in the examination of human eyes.

A fundus camera consists of a light source, a viewing microscope, and a mechanical supporting arrangement that allows precise positioning of the light source and microscope relative to the patient to enable focusing and visualization of the light on selected portions of the patient's eye in order to perform photography. One non-limiting fundus camera that can be used with the present invention is manufactured by Topcon Inc. of Japan.

In Fig. 8.3, non-limiting details of one embodiment for the electrical components used in this device are seen.

In still another embodiment, the described device may be incorporated with another device used in ophthalmology, such as, but not limited to, an Ocular Coherence Tomography (OCT) machine, that can provide the incident light and focusing on the eye necessary to the performance of the method.

In another embodiment, the operation of the device or devices may be automated, such that an operator is not required to make the measurements.

Correlator 265 counts for a predetermined time interval and performs a well-known mathematical operation to obtain the correlation function. A suitable time interval can be approximately 2 µs though another measurement duration may be selected by experimentation. The sample time may be chosen to further characterize the population of light scatters. Measurements taken at shorter sample times, i.e., at 1.5 µs, appear to be more characteristic of smaller and/or faster scattering elements whereas measurements made at longer sample times, i.e., 200 µs, appear more characteristic of larger and/or slower scattering elements. Multiple measurements may be taken and the results averaged to minimize artifacts.

The correlator utilizes the received counts to solve the following equation for the autocorrelation function $C_m(t)$:

$$C_m(t) = \sum_{i=1}^{i=n} p_i p_i + m$$

where

t = the length of the predetermined time interval
i = an index number whose range is one to the total number of intervals
p_i = the number of pulses occurring during the ith time interval
n = the total number of intervals
m = an integer whose range is the number of correlator channels

In accordance with the above equation, correlator 270 produces solutions or points (one for each value of m) in a time sequence, each measurement separated by the value of t. These measurements may be plotted against time to produce a curve that may then be displayed for examination on a personal computer monitor.

More specifically, the program calculates the first and second cumulants (and their respective statistical uncertainties) of the decay rate distribution from a weighted-least-squares fit of the measured autocorrelation function. Calculations are performed using the results of the cumulants analysis to yield the average translational diffusion coefficient, effective diameter and in certain instances, the average molecular weight.

For the simplest case of monodisperse particles, the field correlation is a single decaying exponential. If the polydispersity is not too great, the field autocorrelation function is nearly exponential. Two parameters that are frequently used to characterize particle distribution are the average decay rate and the polydispersity parameter.

The diffusion coefficient (D) is also related to the correlation function $C_m(t)$ determined by the correlator by the following equation:

$$C_m(t) = A + Be^{-2DK2m(t)}$$

where

A, B = constants dependent on the physical details of the measurement
K = the scattering constant for the eye which is $4\pi/\lambda$ (sin $\theta/2$) where λ is the wavelength and θ is the scattering angle
t = the length of the predetermined time interval
m = an integer whose range is the number of correlator channels

Therefore, the values of the diffusion coefficient D and the constants A and B in the above equation can be determined, with the aid of computer, from the autocorrelation curve produced by the correlator 265 by using standard curve fitting and analysis techniques. The calculated diffusion coefficient, the average decay rate, the polydispersity parameters, the statistical uncertainties of each of these parameters and other calculated mathematical terms including the effective diameter and molecular weight, can be stored in the computer along with other patient data.

The apparatus shown in Figs. 8.1 and 8.2 is used to perform a measurement as follows: with a patient sitting at the fundus camera, the operator sets up the device in the same way that the device would be set up during a normal ophthalmic procedure to take a fundus photograph. In order to measure various positions within the retina or choroid, it may be necessary that the pupil be dilated using routinely available dilating drops as normally used during the course of a complete ophthalmic evaluation.

The illumination light of the fundus camera is used to focus the laser beam on the desired spot on the retina. The illumination beam is turned off when the measurement is made. An infrared system may be used to aid in the maintenance of the light beam at the measurement site during the time the fundus camera illumination light is off.

In order to accurately compare measurements made from an individual with measurements made from the same individual at a later time or with measurements from a different individual, the compared measurements could be made from approximately the same position in the retina. Measurements obtained from other positions in the retina may give somewhat different results, which can provide additional information concerning the health of the patient.

At the present time, vascular endothelial growth factor inhibitors are injected into the vitreous cavity of patient's eyes to treat neovascular or "wet" age-related macular degeneration. Using the above system, preliminary results have demonstrated that the average decay constant, or Gamma, decreases immediately following injection. It appears that successful treatment resulting in the resolution of subretinal fluid and a decrease in leakage results in an increase in Gamma, and unsuccessful treatment does not, and that eyes receiving multiple injections of some of these types of drugs may exhibit lower measurements than the fellow, untreated eye which may have future negative consequences on the health of the eye.

Patients undergoing retinal or optic nerve stem cell surgery have been tested using this system. A measurement is made from the posterior pole of the retina the day before surgery, and the patient is remeasured at 3 months and 6 months postoperatively. Preliminary data indicates that though there may not be any visible changes by fundus photography or OCT in those patients with improved vision after the stem cell surgery, the postoperative diffusion coefficient is greater than the preoperative measurement. Those patients whom did not experience an improvement in vision after the stem cell surgery did not demonstrate a change in the diffusion coefficient postoperatively.

All locations, sizes, shapes, measurements, amounts, angles, voltages, frequencies, component or part locations, configurations, temperatures, weights, dimensions, values, time periods, percentages, materials, orientations, etc. discussed above or shown in the drawings are merely by way of example and are not considered limiting and other locations, sizes, shapes, measurements, amounts, angles, voltages, frequencies, component or part locations, configurations, temperatures, weights, dimensions, values, time periods, percentages, materials, orientations, etc. can be chosen and used and all are considered within the scope of the invention. Dimensions of certain parts as shown in the drawings may have been modified and/

or exaggerated for the purpose of clarity of illustration and are not considered limiting.

Changes and modifications within the spirit and scope of the invention will be apparent to those skilled in ophthalmology. It is expected that advancements in electronics will simplify the design of this system. The diffusion coefficient can be replaced by another measure such as the decay constant. The essential point is that variations in the intensity of the back-scattered light are the basis of the measurement. That measurement may then be utilized to obtain derivatives. The form in which those variations are presented is mainly a matter of individual preference. Such obvious modifications and changes are intended to be covered by the appended claims.

Unless feature(s), part(s), component(s), characteristic(s), or function(s) described in the specification or shown in the drawings for a claim element, claim step, or claim term specifically appear in the claim with the claim element, claim step, or claim term, then the inventor does not consider such feature(s), part(s), component(s), characteristic(s), or function(s) to be included for the claim element, claim step, or claim term in the claim for examination purposes and when and if the claim element, claim step, or claim term is interpreted or construed. Similarly, with respect to any "means for" elements in the claims, the inventor considers such language to require only the minimal amounts of features, components, steps, or parts from the specification to achieve the function of the "means for" language and not all of the features, components, steps, or parts describe in the specification that are related to the function of the "means for" language.

While the invention has been described and disclosed in certain terms and has disclosed certain embodiments or modifications, persons skilled in the art who have acquainted themselves with the invention, will appreciate that it is not necessarily limited by such terms, nor to the specific embodiments and modification disclosed herein. Thus, a wide variety of alternatives, suggested by the teachings herein, can be practiced without departing from the spirit of the invention, and rights to such alternatives are particularly reserved and considered within the scope of the invention.

What is claimed is:

Claims

1. A method for aiding in detecting the beginning or early onset of a medical condition by calculation of a diffusion coefficient from a retina or choroid of a patient's in vivo eye, comprising the steps as follows:

   (a) Directing a beam of light from a low-power laser or other coherent light source at a spot in the retina or choroid of the patient's eye.
   (b) Measuring the fluctuations in the intensity of the back-scattered light.

(c) Comparing the measure fluctuations results from step (b) with previously obtained measurements results taken from the retina or choroid of one or more normal or disease-free patients of a similar age to an age of the patient.

2. The method for aiding in detecting of claim 1 wherein the previously obtained measurements taken from the retina or choroid of the one or more normal or disease-free patients establishes a plurality of normal or disease-free measurements.
3. The method for aiding in detecting of claim 2 further comprising the step of storing the plurality of normal or disease-free measurements in an electronic database prior to performing step (a) on the patient's eye.
4. The method for aiding in detecting of claim 1 further comprising the step of periodically repeating steps (a) and (b) for the patient; and determining any changes in measurements for the patient based on measurements taken before and after a therapeutic intervention for the patient.
5. The method for aiding in detecting of claim 1 further comprising the step of diagnosing a disease for the patient, measuring a severity of a diagnosed disease, monitoring for progress and treatment of a medical condition, or assessing an efficacy of a therapeutic intervention using a diffusion coefficient.
6. The method for detecting of claim 1 further comprising the step of using or comparing an obtained measurement with an Ocular Coherence Tomography (OCT) image and measurement that was also made from the same or nearby area of a retina.
7. The method for detecting of claim 1 wherein the medical condition is dementia.
8. A method for obtaining a measurement from a retina of a patient that is used as an aide in detecting the beginning or early onset of a medical condition for the patient comprising the following steps:

(a) Taking a fundus photograph for a patient using a fundus camera.
(b) Obtaining one or more measurements from the fundus photograph.
(c) Comparing the obtained measurements for the patient with prior measurements made for the patient or prior measurements from a different individual.

9. The method for obtaining a measurement of claim 8 wherein the measurements obtained in step (b) and the prior measurements for the patient or from the different individual are taken approximately at a same position of a human retina.
10. The method for obtaining a measurement of claim 9 wherein the measurement obtained in step (b) is made from a posterior pole of the patient's retina a day before surgery for the patient.
11. The method for obtaining a measurement of claim 10 wherein steps (a) and (b) are periodically repeated post-surgery for use in step (c).
12. The method for obtaining a measurement of claim 8 further comprising the step of dilating the pupil and the one or more measurements are a plurality of measurements of various positions within the patient's retina or choroid.

13. The method for obtaining a measurement of claim 8 further comprising the steps of directing a beam of light from a low-power laser or other coherent light source at a sport in the retina or choroid of the patient's eye and focusing the beam of light using an illumination light of the fundus camera.

14. The method for obtaining a measurement of claim 13 further comprising the step of turning the illumination light of the fundus camera off prior to taking the measurement.

15. The method for obtaining a measurement of claim 14 further comprising the step of using an infrared viewing light to aid in the maintenance of the light beam at a measurement site during a time period that the fundus camera illumination light is off during a measurement performance.

16. The method for obtaining a measurement of claim 8 further comprising the step of choosing a location for taking the measurement at the patient's retina or choroid on the basis of fundus autofluorescence, fundus fluorescein angiography, OCT, or another imaging technology.

17. The method for obtaining a measurement of claim 8 further comprising the step detecting fluctuations in intensities of back-scattered light using a digital photon counter.

18. The method for obtaining a measurement of claim 17 further comprising the steps processing an output of the digital photon counter using a digital correlator and providing a set of numbers for use in calculating a diffusion coefficient.

19. A method for aiding in the detection of a medical disease, including dementia and retinal conditions, through ascertaining and studying a diffusion coefficient of tissue for a patient, comprising the following steps:

   (a) Directing light from a laser or other coherent light source at a patient's retina or choroid.

   (b) Measuring fluctuations in intensity of back-scattered light caused by the movement of light scatterers in the tissue.

   (c) Comparing measurements obtained in step (b) to normal measurements stored in a database or to previous measurements obtained for the patient.

   (d) Based on the comparison in step (c) in combination with an eye examination and an OCT image/measurement, ascertaining if there have been any changes to the medical disease or the effectiveness of any therapy being given to the patient for the medical disease.

Bibliography

Weiss JN. Laser light scattering of in-vivo human lenses. Am J Ophthalmol. 1982;94:683.

Weiss JN. Laser device seen as aid to early detection of cataracts. Ophthalmol Times. 1982;1:1.

Weiss JN. New laser technique detects eye disease. Joslin Diabet Center Newsl. 1983;11(4):8.

Weiss JN, Rand LI, Gleason RE, Soeldner JS. Laser light scattering spectroscopy of in-vivo human lenses. Invest Ophthalmol Vis Sci. 1984;25:594–8.

Nishio I, Weiss JN, Tanaka T, Clark JI, Giblin FJ, Reddy VN, Benedek GB. In-vivo observation of lens protein diffusivity in normal and X-irradiated rabbit lenses. Exp Eye Res. 1984;39:61–8.

Bursell SE, Weiss JN, Eichold BH. Diagnostic Laser light scattering spectroscopy for human eyes. Proc Int Congr Appl Laser Electro Opt. 1984;43:61–7.

Weiss JN, Bursell SE, Gleason RE, Eichold BH. Photon correlation spectroscopy of in-vivo human cornea. Cornea. 1986;5(1):19–24.

Bursell SE, Baker RS, Weiss JN, Haughton JF, Rand LI. Clinical photon correlation spectroscopy evaluation of human diabetic lenses. Exp Eye Res. 1989;49:241–58.

Bursell SE, Karalekas DP, Craig MS. The effect of acute changes in blood glucose on lenses in diabetic and non-diabetic subjects using quasi-elastic light scattering spectroscopy. Curr Eye Res. 1989;8:821–34. Bursell SE, Weiss JN, Karalekas DP, Craig MS. Correction Notice. Curr Eye Res. 1992;11(5):479

Chu B. Laser light scattering. New York: Academic; 1974.

Koppel DE. Analysis of macromolecular polydispersity in intensity correlation spectroscopy: the method of cumulants. J Chem Phys. 1972;57:4814–20.

Weiss JN, Benes SC, Levy S. Stem Cell Ophthalmology Treatment Study: bone marrow derived stem cells in the treatment of non-arteritic ischemic optic neuropathy (NAION). Stem Cell Invest. 2017;4:94. http://sci.amegroups.com/issue/view/632

© The Editor(s) (if applicable) and The Author(s), under exclusive license to
Springer Nature Switzerland AG 2022
J. N. Weiss, *Dynamic Light Scattering Spectroscopy of the Human Eye*,
https://doi.org/10.1007/978-3-031-06624-5

Index

Printed in the United States
by Baker & Taylor Publisher Services